Called Through Cancer

Called Through Cancer

Vocation, Vulnerability and the God Who Holds Us

Lisa Barnett

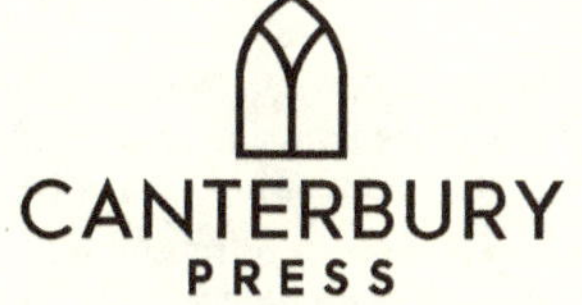

First published in 2026 by Canterbury Press

Editorial office
3rd Floor, Invicta House
110 Golden Lane,
London EC1Y 0TG, UK
www.canterburypress.co.uk

Canterbury Press is an imprint of Hymns Ancient & Modern Ltd
(a registered charity)

HYMNS Ancient & Modern

Hymns Ancient & Modern® is a registered trademark of
Hymns Ancient & Modern Ltd
13A Hellesdon Park Road, Norwich,
Norfolk NR6 5DR, UK

British Library Cataloguing in Publication data

A catalogue record for this book is available
from the British Library

ISBN: 978 1 78622 746 1

EU GPSR Authorised Representative
LOGOS EUROPE, 9 rue Nicolas Poussin, 17000, LA ROCHELLE, France
E-mail: Contact@logoseurope.eu

Typeset by Regent Typesetting

Contents

Introduction vii

1 Calling 1
2 Called to tussle with suffering 9
3 Called to face the darkness 17
4 Called to vulnerability 27
5 Called to community 35
6 An embodied calling 45
7 Called to be ready to die 53
8 Called to a new normal 63

Afterword 71
Study Guide 75
References and Further Reading 81

Introduction

A week after the second dose of a very tough chemotherapy regime, I was seeing a friend. I had discovered that during this fortnightly chemo I would only have three good days when I was feeling well enough to see anyone. As we sat and chatted, she asked me if I was finding it hard not to be living out my vocation as a priest and vicar while I went through cancer treatment. I'd been ordained for 17 years; so it was a good question. I thought about it for a moment and recognized from within myself an unexpected answer. I took a deep breath, and tried to explain that it felt OK, because I knew that this journey through cancer was my vocation for this season. I saw the surprise on her face, as she contemplated the idea that I could use the words 'cancer' and 'vocation' in the same sentence. Yet I knew that what I had just told her was a deep, God-given truth. That conversation stayed with me, and has become the inspiration for this book.

Everyone's experience with cancer will be unique, both because of the specific histology of the cancer and its recommended treatments, and because of the circumstances of the cancer patient. I was diagnosed with lobular breast cancer, which had spread to the nearby lymph nodes. Each day in the UK, 22 women are diagnosed with lobular breast cancer, but it is under-researched and consequently lacks appropriate treatment options.

My treatment involved a mastectomy and lymph node clearance, chemotherapy, radiotherapy, and then several long-term medications (for between two and ten years) aimed at preventing the cancer from recurring. My home life when I was diagnosed was with my husband, eleven-year-old twin daughters and eight-year-old son, and I served as a team rector in West Sussex, based primarily at the large town-centre church of St Mary's, Horsham.

Whatever has brought you to exploring this book, you are known and loved by God. I pray that, through my reflections, you might find hope for your journey, and might be drawn closer to the God of hope, who has reminded me again through my cancer journey that in life and in death, in illness and in suffering, I am held in him.

I

Calling

As a teenager and a new Christian, I still remember the zeal and energy with which I explored the question of what God wanted me to do with my life. My deep longing was to give all I had to serve the God who had, in the words spoken to me by the bishop at my confirmation, called me by name and made me his own. My longing was reflected in 'The Summer Day' by the poet Mary Oliver:

> Tell me, what is it you plan to do
> with your one wild and precious life?

In those youthful days, discerning God's will felt vital and complex, shaped by an unspoken fear that, by making the wrong decision about what A levels to take or which university course to apply for, I might somehow miss God's will, and end up on completely the wrong path. During that intense and emotive time, I still recall the pithy words of a Church Army Evangelist, Andrew Perry, when he came to visit the Christian Union at our sixth-form college, and told us: 'God is more concerned about who you are than where you are, and guidance is about knowing the Guide.'

These words became a vital bedrock for my ongoing exploration of how I might live my life for God and ensured that, as I explored my vocation, I never lost sight of the primacy of my relationship with God.

As the years went on, I became more confident that God was inviting me to serve him through ordained ministry, even though

I was young and female, and most of the priests that I knew were older and male. As I tussled with my growing sense of calling, I was reminded that my vocation was about being true to all that God had created in me, rather than trying to squeeze myself into a vicar-shaped box, as Parker Palmer articulates well:

> Vocation does not come from a voice 'out there' calling me to become something I am not. It comes from a voice 'in here' calling me to be the person I was born to be, to fulfil the original selfhood given me at birth by God. (Palmer, *Let your Life Speak*)

It was significant that the moment I felt most conscious of God calling me to be ordained was in the emotionally bruised time when I arrived home from my Church Mission Society gap year, where I had been working with the Orthodox Church in Russia. It had been a challenging time, practically, theologically, spiritually, and there was much to process when I returned home. It was as I sat in church, so aware of my brokenness, and brought all the complexity of the experience to God, that I was most conscious of God speaking into my heart: 'I'm calling you to be ordained. I'm not calling you because you've got your theology all sorted, or because you're strong or competent. I'm calling you, because I'm calling you, because I'm calling you. This is who I've made you to be.'

In the inevitable moments of impostor syndrome in the subsequent years that I've served in ordained ministry, I am often drawn back to that moment of brokenness, when God made clear that his call was not dependent on my particular gifts or skills, but on his call and faithfulness. As I went through the Church of England's vocation processes, with their helpful reminder that our vocation is not just about our own sense of God's call, but also the discernment and needs of the church, I found myself articulating with increasing nuance the particular way that I sensed God inviting me to inhabit Anglican priesthood. It was about being a catalyst to enable the church to be the church more fully, supporting and encouraging the people of God to be ambassadors for Christ and a channel for God's love in the world. I valued the words attributed to St Catherine of Siena: 'Be who you were made to be and you will set the world on fire.' I increasingly understood my own vocation as supporting each Christian to find their unique way of being all that God had created them to be.

Serving as a priest in God's church has been full of joy, privilege and a deep sense that this is indeed what God has made me for. Yet I've never felt that priesthood was my only vocation. Meeting my husband during my curacy, I was delighted to be called to become a wife and, a couple of years later, a mother. Over the years, I've had the privilege of establishing and leading gospel choirs and a community choir, and I've loved offering my musical skills into this further vocation as a choir director. I have also been deeply involved in vocations work, as both an assistant diocesan director of ordinands and a national advisor for bishops' panels, supporting those exploring ordained ministry. I've supported three curates through their curacies, and nurtured two new Readers into active ministry, and each of these things has been a huge privilege. These are all things that I can put on my CV, and they have been vocations that have brought me great joy. But at my deepest place, I still consider that my primary vocation is as a child of God and a disciple of Christ.

Recognizing and naming this primary vocation really matters, because, without it, there is a risk that we end up restricting the language of vocation to clergy, monks and nuns, or those offering formal, licensed ministry within the church. When Mary Oliver asks us what we are going to do with our one wild and precious life, I don't think she expected us all to answer by talking about what we do in church. In the contemporary church there is a renewed commitment to inviting all Christians to acknowledge the vocation that springs from our baptism, reinforced by the Church of England's provocative report, *Setting God's People Free*:

> Both clergy and laity are baptised disciples and live out our calling together. Lay people – like clergy – have vocations and callings. They just happen to be callings and vocations which do not require ordination. (p. 4)

At a baptism, candidates are commissioned using these or similar words: 'In baptism God invites you on a lifelong journey. Together with all God's people you must explore the way of Jesus and grow in friendship with God, in love for his people, and in serving others.' As we use these words of commissioning with baptism candidates of all ages, we have no idea what vocations God might call them into through the years. We hope and pray that, through the gift of baptism, God will nurture the faith and grow the unique vocations of each person so that in school, in their career, in their voluntary work, in the way they handle their money, their time, their relationships, in their words and their choices, they might continue to love, serve and follow Christ. As St Paul wrote to the church community in Colossae, 'Whatever you do, whether in word or deed, do it all in the name of the Lord Jesus, giving thanks to God the Father through him' (Colossians 3.17).

As Christians today, we share in the overarching vocation to all God's people through the generations: to be loved and to love. We are called to receive the generous, gracious and forgiving love of God, and then to be a channel of that love in the world. Just as Jesus called the first disciples to follow him, so he continues to make that call through the centuries in a way that is both universal and personal, and both lifelong and unique to each conversation, encounter and choice.

As we grow as Christians, we will continue to be aware of our sinfulness and frailty, as St Paul expresses it in the Letter to the Romans: 'For I have the desire to do what is good, but I cannot carry it out. For I do not do the good I want to do, but the evil I do not want to do – this I keep on doing' (Romans 7.18–19). Yet we are also given the extraordinary privilege of being filled with the indwelling Holy Spirit and participating in God's redeeming work, as ambassadors of his love, and in the bringing in of God's kingdom: 'For we are God's handiwork, created in Christ Jesus to do good works, which God prepared in advance for us to do' (Ephesians 2.10). This vocation doesn't require us to complete any course or pass any test, and we will regularly get things wrong as we seek to live it out. But we won't be sacked, or kicked out, or stepped down, because this calling rests on God's gracious invitation and our response, however tentative, of faith and service.

Sometimes our vocational journey will require extended times of discernment, supported by Christian friends and the wider church, as we consider stepping into vocations that will involve big changes to our working patterns and family life. But some vocations will be discerned in the moment, as we sense the Spirit of God prompting us to buy some lunch for a homeless person that we pass in town, or to take some time to pop in on an elderly neighbour that we haven't seen for a while. Each of these actions are moments of vocation, moments when we are responding to the invitation of the Holy Spirit to be vehicles of God's love in the world.

As we each respond to the call of Christ in each moment, sometimes this will mean offering our gifts, skills and competencies, and finding joy in ministering according to our 'sweet spot'. Sometimes our service will be shaped by a need within our communities, and the gentle prompting of God in our hearts that perhaps we might be the one who could respond, even if our service will be uncomfortable and costly, even if it means bringing our weakness rather than our strength.

The prophets of the Old Testament, who are often called to challenge God's wayward people to return to God, remind us that our vocations will not always be easy. Jeremiah is often known as the depressed prophet, and has an especially difficult time:

> I am ridiculed all day long; everyone mocks me. Whenever I speak, I cry out proclaiming violence and destruction. So the

> word of the Lord has brought me insult and reproach all day long. (Jeremiah 20.7–8)

Jeremiah recognizes that his prophetic ministry is his vocation even though it's difficult. It is such a deep part of who he is that he can't run away from it, though he may want to: 'But if I say, "I will not mention him or speak any more in his name," his word is in my heart like a fire, a fire shut up in my bones' (Jeremiah 20.9).

Inspired by St Paul's image of the church as a body in 1 Corinthians, we are invited to explore the particular parts that we are called to play at different times in our lives, aware that sometimes the Spirit will prompt us to say 'no' to vocations that aren't ours:

> If the whole body were an eye, where would the sense of hearing be? If the whole body were an ear, where would the sense of smell be? But in fact God has placed the parts in the body, every one of them, just as he wanted them to be. (1 Corinthians 12.17–18)

When Adam and Eve ate the fruit of the tree of knowledge in the garden of Eden, they were enticed by the thought of becoming something that they weren't called to be and becoming like God (Genesis 2—3). We must guard against a temptation to want to play parts in God's kingdom that are not ours to play. Being at peace with vocations that aren't ours as well as those that are is a daily challenge, and one that requires us to learn to listen carefully to the promptings of the Holy Spirit.

It is vital that the vocation of Christians is never limited to the way we serve within our church communities. As important as it is that our churches have enough people to be welcomers, to lead home groups, to serve on refreshment rotas and tech teams, we should have as much expectation of God being at work in us and through us on Monday morning as we do on Sunday at church. One of the core tenets of Ignatian spirituality is the invitation to find God in all things. This springs from the belief of St Ignatius of Loyola (1491–1556) that God's presence can be found in every aspect of life, and not just in religious settings. Western society encourages us to compartmentalize between our spiritual life, professional life and personal life, but the Bible sees no such distinction. As Christian minister and author Tyler Staton preached to his church, Bridgetown, in Portland, Oregon:

> The Biblical story is one that gets worked out and expressed in the material world and permeates every area of our lives. So to live as disciples of Christ means to eat meals, budget, go to work, raise children, hang out with friends, make weekend plans, and do it all marching to the beat of a different king in the procession of another kingdom. (Staton, 'Vocation')

At St Mary's, Horsham, a couple of years ago, we enjoyed hearing from members of our congregation each Sunday morning about their TTT: This Time Tomorrow. Each person shared with us what they would be doing on Monday morning, and how their Christian faith was worked out during the six days of the week that they weren't in church. We heard from an architect and a foster mum, a nurse and someone who was retired. Each story reminded us of the diverse places that church members were spending their lives, and the unique opportunities and challenges that they each had in order to live distinctive lives as children of God and disciples of Christ.

Brother Lawrence spent much of his life washing dishes in a monastery in seventeenth-century Paris. This was the context in which he learnt to be with and in God in each moment of his life, and not just when at prayer in the chapel. In the compilation of his writings, *The Practice of the Presence of God*, it is said of him:

> Everything was the same to him, every place, every task. The good Brother found God everywhere, as much while he was repairing shoes as while he was praying with the community.

> He was not eager to go into retreat, for he found in his common tasks the same God to worship as in the depths of the deserts. (Brother Lawrence, *The Practice of the Presence of God*, p. 88)

Though I wasn't expecting 2025 to bring me a new vocation, when cancer became part of my story, I nonetheless recognized that this was God's vocation for me for this season. Naming the cancer journey as my vocation ensured that I lived with God in each moment, rather than seeing the cancer treatment as something to get through as quickly as possible, so that I could get back to my *real* vocation. Allowing the treatment to be vocational brought a deep sense of freedom, but also of hopeful expectation of all that God would do in me and through me as I faced it. As Tyler Staton, who himself had serious cancer during 2024, expresses it: 'You can meet God in a deeper way in circumstances you'd never choose' (Staton, 'Ask, Seek, Knock').

As the days, weeks and months of treatment progressed, I kept returning to the Ignatian questions: 'What is God's call to me in this season of cancer treatment, and how am I being invited to find God in this difficult time?' I kept holding onto God's lifelong invitation to an ever-deeper surrender and trust of all that I am and have to God. Though I was scared at what the journey might bring, I was also confident that God would be with me through it; calling me and leading me.

2

Called to tussle with suffering

It had already been an intense morning. Up at 7am, doing the school drop-off at 8.15am, then heading straight off to one of the local hospitals. I should have been in plenty of time for a 10am appointment, but there had been problems with flooding on the road, and I found myself stuck in one traffic jam after another. I ended up running into the hospital at 10am exactly, desperately scanning the different signs to work out where I should be going, and then muttering apologetically to the staff member at the desk.

I'd gone to the hospital on my own. I knew it would be a long day and I was familiar with the processes. I'd been through this twice before, finding something suspicious and being referred to the hospital for checks. I was happy enough to let the process run its course; I had a novel to enjoy, and there's always plenty of people-watching to keep me entertained in a hospital.

I bought a couple of snacks from the hospital shop and waited for my name to be called. First a nurse took down the details of the referral and conducted her own assessment. It was obvious that she thought there was something concerning; so I was sent on to a second waiting room, ready to be called for a mammogram. Some young parents joined me in the waiting room with a tiny newborn baby who needed some kind of scan. Wondering about their story, I found myself reflecting that I was so grateful that it was me who was facing this medical issue, rather than one of my children. I whispered a quick prayer for the newborn, and the anxious parents.

After the mammogram, I was called into a third room and invited up onto the hospital bed, where a friendly doctor did an ultrasound and then confirmed that she'd need to do some biopsies, too. It was during the biopsies that I discovered that I'm really good at bleeding! Though I couldn't see what was happening, there were several rapid dashes for paper towels to try to mop up the blood, regular questions ('Are you sure you're not on blood thinners?') and general warm laughter that it was probably good that I couldn't see what I looked like!

Then the moment came, as I lay on the hospital bed, I asked the kind doctor the direct question: 'Do you think it's cancer?'

'Yes,' she answered, looking at me sympathetically, and I was so grateful for her honesty. That was the moment when I began my new and difficult vocation, as a cancer patient.

A couple of months later, I was recovering from my mastectomy, the first stage of my treatment, when our lovely cleaner, Catherine, arrived and asked how I was doing. She then looked at me directly, and acknowledged that she'd been worrying over the weekend about whether my cancer had rocked my faith. She was really disturbed at the possibility that it might have done, and that I might need to stop being a vicar. I was so touched by her concern, and reminded again of the responsibility of being a public figure of faith during times of suffering.

None of us knows how we will respond when we, or a close family member, face a serious health issue. However much we have a carefully thought-out theology of suffering, we are compelled to revisit it when the suffering becomes a personal experience. In trying to make sense of what we're facing, we can find ourselves looking for someone or something to blame, whether it's the NHS processes, some kind of societal cause or God. We may even find ourselves wondering if our suffering is a punishment. As Christians, we sometimes harbour an unspoken but deeply rooted idea that our faith should be a kind of divine insurance policy, that if we're good people we should somehow be protected from the suffering of the world.

When the wife of Australian pastor Mark Sayers was diagnosed with serious cancer, a lot of people said that they couldn't believe it had happened to a pastor. Sayers reflects that in a lot of churches, 'there's almost been an implicit prosperity Gospel, of the pastor who's got their entire life together' (Staton, 'Healing, with Mark Sayers'). Yet none of us is immune from suffering in this life, and that includes Christians and Christian ministers. What makes the experience unique for the minister is the responsibility to try to be an example and a role model in following Christ even through suffering. Christian ministers will regularly be invited to a precious journey of walking with others through their experience of suffering, and so how ministers make that journey will end up being an example to others.

Jewish society in Jesus' day drew causal links between a person's experience of suffering and their sin. We see this in John 9, when the disciples ask: 'Rabbi, who sinned, this man or his parents, that he was born blind?' Jesus challenges this perspective firmly, responding, 'Neither this man nor his parents sinned.' On another occasion, when Jesus is told of the suffering of some Galileans whose blood Pilate had mixed with their animal sacrifices, Jesus responds: 'Do you think that these Galileans were worse sinners than all the other Galileans because they suffered this way? I tell you, no!' (Luke 13.2–3).

A vocation to suffering is the universal experience of humanity, as we live in our fallen and broken world, but acknowledging that truth doesn't make it any easier to live with. As I made my way through the initial numb phase after my diagnosis and began to tussle with this vocation to suffering, I was surprised to realize that I didn't find myself nursing a refrain of 'it's not fair!' Perhaps because I have been aware of being blessed during my life, perhaps because in ministry I have walked alongside many who have suffered in different ways, I actually felt 'why not me?' And having worked through the initial shock, I found myself being given a renewed confidence that in life and in death I belong to God. I found comfort from the words of Julian of Norwich, the fourteenth-century mystic, who wrote, 'If there is anywhere on earth a lover of God who is always kept safe, I know nothing of it, for it was not shown to me. But this was shown: that in falling and rising again we are always kept in that same precious love' (Julian of Norwich, *Revelations of Divine Love*).

However, recognizing the trauma that my cancer would cause for my family and children, and trusting God's goodness and care for them, was much, much harder. Trusting God to provide for the children if I died young was the hardest part of my own tussling with suffering. That Holy Week, I was particularly conscious of Jesus' worry for his loved ones, and his words from the cross, asking John to take Mary as his own mother, and asking Mary to take John as her son (John 19.26–7).

A friend from my previous parish, Jade, sent me such a moving message:

> I want to stamp my foot, Lisa, and shout, 'This isn't fair,' but when Mikey was in hospital, and we spoke a bit about my mum dying young of cancer and about Mikey being poorly, you said, 'God gets sad about these things, too,' and that helps me through things more than you could know.

It was so beautiful to hear her reflecting back to me the simple words that I'd shared with her when her young son was born prematurely, about the sadness that God also feels about suffering.

Reflecting on a vocation to suffering, the intriguing Book of Job becomes especially poignant. The story opens with Job as a man very blessed with family, livestock and herds, and a man of deep faith and trust in God. We see God delighting in Job, boasting about the way that he lives out his life and his faith. Satan appears before the throne of God, and challenges God that Job only trusts him because he is blessed. So God gives Satan permission to remove some of Job's blessings and Job loses his flocks, his herds and his children. Yet he responds with a remarkable declaration of faith and surrender: 'The Lord gave and the Lord has taken away: May the name of the Lord be praised' (Job 1.21).

Satan approaches God a second time, again posing the challenge that Job is still only trusting God because he has kept his health and, again, God gives Satan permission to remove Job's health as well. In Chapter 2, Job is afflicted with painful sores from the soles of his feet to the top of his head and is described as scraping himself with broken pottery as he sits among the ashes. His wife goads him, 'Are you still holding on to your integrity? Curse God and die!' But Job responds, 'Shall we accept good from God and not trouble?' (Job 2. 9–10).

Though the Book of Job doesn't try to provide every answer to the challenges of suffering, it does make it clear that God allows suffering but doesn't create it. In order to speak of a vocation to suffering, it is important to be clear that God hasn't sent suffering to any of us in order to punish us. The experience of suffering is common to all of humanity, but it can become a vocation if we allow God to journey with us through it, reminded of St Ignatius's expectation that we can find God in every moment.

As the Book of Job continues, we see its eponymous character wrestling with God about what has happened to him. He begins to find words to express his grief and pain, and his questions become more direct and raw. Pete Greig reflects that the Bible is much more honest about suffering than the church is, and we see it laid out vividly in the Book of Job (Staton, 'Ask, Seek, Knock').

In his biography of C. S. Lewis, Alister McGrath explains that Lewis had written *The Problem of Pain* in his younger years, as a largely theoretical and academic exercise. McGrath comments:

> Suffering can only be little more than a logical riddle for those who encounter it from a safe distance. When it is experienced firsthand, as when Lewis lost his mother, and again at the devastating death of Davidman, it is like an emotional battering ram, crashing into the gates of the castle of faith. (McGrath, *C. S. Lewis: A Life*)

The death of his beloved wife Joy Davidman, after only four years of marriage, prompted Lewis to write *A Grief Observed*. The book takes the form of a series of journal entries, as Lewis seeks to use words to process his overwhelming grief, and as he boldly speaks out loud his most desolate moments and experiences:

> Where is God? ... go to him when your need is desperate, when all other help is in vain, and what do you find? A door slammed in your face and the sound of bolting and double bolting on the inside. After that, silence. (Lewis, *A Grief Observed*)

Instead of seeking to defend God from the accusations of a suffering world, Lewis's book articulates with extraordinary honesty the experience of a mature believer who faces their own overwhelming time of suffering. Having written numerous books as a gifted creative writer and theologian, Lewis now uses a different voice of profound authenticity and depth as he shares his honest and heartfelt struggle with God.

In times of suffering, we're invited to join C. S. Lewis in bringing to God our honest, heartfelt prayers, including our anger for the moments when God seems absent. God is big enough for our pain and our questions, however unpalatable they may feel, and God is big enough for all our emotions, however scared we might be to recognize and name them. Learning to tussle with God during times of suffering is not always easy. Some of us have learnt to adopt a 'prayer voice' of reverence and obedience, and can feel uncomfortable about the idea of speaking out words of rage, disappointment and bitterness to God in prayer. One way of beginning to do this could be using the Imprecatory Psalms, sometimes known as the Psalms of Anger. In Psalm 13, David cries out to God:

> How long, O Lord? Will you forget me forever? How long will you hide your face from me? How long must I wrestle with my thoughts and day after day have sorrow in my heart? How long will my enemy triumph over me? Look on me and answer, Lord my God. (Psalm 13.1–3)

If we don't work through times of suffering honestly with God, there's a risk that we may end up trusting God a little less as we emerge from the suffering, while still churning out the same Christian platitudes about God's love and goodness. This tussling with God may also involve waiting patiently through the long days of struggle for hope to emerge and for God's comfort to be received. As the Psalmist writes, 'Why, my soul, are you downcast, why so disturbed within me? Put your hope in God, for I will *yet* praise him, my saviour and my God' (Psalm 42.11). If, like Job, like the Psalmist, like C. S. Lewis, we can allow our prayer in difficult times to be deep and raw, we open the possibility of a more honest trust in God emerging.

During my cancer journey, I found myself referring on several occasions to my own 'Last Suppers'. These included the Christmas lunch that I shared with the parish Mothers' Union before heading to the hospital to have my cancer confirmed, and the night before some of the hardest doses of chemotherapy. This biblical story came to epitomize the painful weightiness of some of my cancer moments, and so I felt led to use Ignatian meditation to imagine myself in the story of the Last Supper and invite Jesus to speak to me there. This became a profound moment of healing, as I shared with Jesus my own weighty burdens, and he spoke to me with deep empathy about his.

By Chapter 38 of the Book of Job, God speaks to Job, but doesn't give explanations for his suffering. Though we may long for answers to the 'why me, why this time, why this way?' questions of suffering, the Book of Job reminds us that there aren't always answers to be found in this life. Instead, God paints for Job an extraordinary vision of who God is, and a 'God's-eye view' of life and the world. The final chapter of Job sees him being healed and restored, and then making a profound declaration of faith following his encounters with God through his experience of suffering: 'My ears had heard of you, but now my eyes have seen you' (Job 42.5).

Job's experience is brought into the twenty-first century by so many stories of people who have faced their own suffering and tussled with God through it. One who has spoken with power and honesty about suffering and faith is Jane 'Nightbirde' Marczewski, who died of cancer when she was 31. She writes in a poem about nights when she couldn't sleep, and would lie on the bathroom floor, vomiting until she was hollow. From this place, she describes with heart-rending authenticity her relationship with God which involves banging loudly on God's door every day, sometimes greeting God with songs and other times with curses. Jane acknowledges that she can be counted among those who are angry, cynical, offended and hardened, and yet knows that she must also be counted as one of the friends of God because through her suffering she has encountered God in profound and unexpected ways. Jane concludes her poem by reflecting that even when she's not so sick, sometimes she still goes to lie on the bathroom mat to wait for God, and comments, 'If you can't see him, look lower. God is on the bathroom floor.'

3

Called to face the darkness

On a Sunday morning in December 2024, I led a busy Christingle service, knowing that, just a few days later, I would be returning to the hospital to receive the results of the biopsies that would confirm the nature of my cancer. As we held our Christingles aloft in our beautiful church, we proclaimed again the truth from the first chapter of John's Gospel, that Christ's light shines in the darkness, and the darkness has not overcome it (John 1.5). I walked home that day with a sense of peace, that if it was going to be my last Sunday working for a while, it had been a good one to end on. I didn't know quite how much I would be challenged in the darkness of the months ahead to keep trusting that the light of Christ would not be overcome.

Having felt quite resilient about facing the surgery and recovery, the next stage of my treatment was five months of chemotherapy, which felt very daunting. The surgery had felt like a sprint, but the chemotherapy felt like a marathon. I was anxious about how my body would respond to the toxic drugs, what side effects I would face, how ill I would feel for how long, and how I could continue to be 'mum' for the children while my body faced such an onslaught of toxicity.

Tyler Staton's description of chemotherapy puts it very starkly:

> I'm being fed a combination of toxins dangerous enough the nurse has to wrap herself in the medical equivalent of a hazmat suit to handle the plastic bags holding litres of liquid that flow right into my arteries. These drugs are killing me slowly, but thankfully first they're killing the cancer, that's killing me quickly. (Staton, *The Familiar Stranger*, Chapter 11)

We often use the image of darkness to describe fears that we don't want to acknowledge or think about because they are so frightening, and facing chemotherapy was a very dark time for me.

One of my children seemed to be especially worried about it, and kept up a running commentary for us: 'I can't believe you're having chemo in 4 days ...' For myself, I noticed that I wanted to get the chemo started as soon as I could, in order that I might know what side effects I'd face. Though the thought of chemotherapy felt very dark and frightening, I wanted to walk swiftly towards the darkness, to allow it to take a form and shape, recognizing that one of the darkest fears is often that of the unknown.

When we face times of serious illness, the image of darkness can give us a powerful visual language with which to express the deep struggles that we are facing. Our experience of darkness can be physical, emotional and spiritual, and might take the form of physical pain, emotional fear and spiritual desolation. Very often these things all come together, leaving us with a sense of existential darkness on every side.

Darkness and light are frequent themes in Scripture, and almost always carry the clear understanding that light is where God is, and is good, hopeful and joyful, while darkness is negative and is to be avoided. This is put particularly starkly in the First Letter of John: 'God is light; in him there is no darkness at all' (1 John 1.5). Yet the story of the creation of the world reminds us that God created the world from darkness, and that 'God called the light "day", and the darkness he called "night"' (Genesis 1.5). Both light and dark are seen as natural and necessary, with no negative connotation attached to the darkness of the night. In the Gospels, we see that the new creation in Jesus emerges from the darkness of the tomb; so darkness is a prerequisite for the creation and re-creation of all things, including ourselves.

Often, the biblical images of darkness serve to remind us that there is nowhere that God isn't, such as in Psalm 139: 'even the darkness will not be dark to you; the night will shine like the day, for darkness is as light to you' (Psalm 139.12). A further verse tucked into the prophecies of Isaiah points to the unexpected gifts of facing the darkness; gifts that may not ever be found if we insist on remaining in the light: 'I will give you the treasures of darkness and riches hidden in secret places, so that you may know that it is I, the Lord, the God of Israel, who call you by your name' (Isaiah 45.3, NRSV).

As we embrace a vocation to face dark times, we may long for God to bring us into times of light, while finding instead that God wants to give us gifts from the darkness. These gifts may not be immediately apparent, they may take time to emerge, and the waiting can be especially painful.

One of the hardest parts of journeying through dark days is longing to experience God's comforting presence but not always encountering God in the ways that we hope to. Christians through the centuries have testified that sometimes it is precisely during the darkest times of suffering that God seems the most absent. In Mother Teresa's writings, which were made public after her death, she wrote, 'I am told God lives in me – and yet the reality of darkness and coldness and emptiness is so great that nothing touches my soul' (Scott, *The Love That Made Mother Teresa*, Chapter 17).

It can be reassuring during dark times to be reminded that Christians through every generation have faced this experience too. A clergy colleague, Revd Jane Willis, put it beautifully: 'Darkness is well and truly on the map of the experience of the people of God; so when we find ourselves in that place, we know that we haven't fallen off the edge of the map.' Psalm 88 particularly acknowledges the pain of dark times, and concludes with the phrase 'darkness is my closest friend' (Psalm 88.18).

In these times of spiritual darkness, it can be important to do what we can to continue in the spiritual disciplines that have sustained us in easier times. When everything goes dark, it may be important to stay with what we have known to be true in the light, while recognizing that some of the patterns of life will need to be adapted for the new season. It may no longer be possible to attend church regularly, and so we can join the many others at home and in hospitals and care homes, who have come to value the livestreamed services from churches up and down the country. We may not have the concentration to read, but we can listen to Christian audiobooks, worship songs or hymns and the audio Bible, allowing the Spirit to minister to us, choosing to invite God into the darkness. During my long weeks of chemotherapy, I watched the livestream of our church service on a Sunday morning, and then, once our curate, Scott, had finished distributing Holy Communion in church, he brought it down the road to me at the vicarage. He then returned to church ready for the notices and final hymn. I felt quite tearful on occasions receiving communion on my doorstep, apart from yet together with my church family.

As we claim the Bible's promise that there is nothing 'that will be able to separate us from the love of God that is in Christ Jesus our Lord' (Romans 8), we can face the darkness with the confident expectation that God is there, while also acknowledging that in difficult times we may not always be able to discern God's loving presence with us.

St John of the Cross, the sixteenth-century mystic and author of *The Dark Night of the Soul*, encourages the Christian to: 'Live in faith and hope, though it be in darkness, for in this darkness God protects the soul. Cast your care upon God for you are His and He will not forget you.'

During times of serious illness, part of the darkness can be the pain of remembering the vibrant communities that continue on without us. We can so easily experience FOMO – 'Fear Of Missing Out'. Yet, if we can receive this restricted time as both gift and vocation, we are invited to rediscover who we are when we're not busy. Eugene Peterson writes about the temptations of defining ourselves by our busyness: 'I want to appear important and significant. What better way than to be busy? The incredible hours, the crowded schedule, and the heavy demands on my time are proof to myself – and to all who will notice – that I am important' (Peterson, *The Contemplative Pastor*).

Times of extended silence and solitude also compel us to face up to parts of ourselves that we may prefer to avoid. As we work through these uncomfortable revelations, we are invited to find a deeper peace, both with ourselves and with God. In our noisy society, it's easy to find ever more effective strategies to avoid silence, and equally easy to presume that this is a twenty-first-century problem. Yet 400 years ago Blaise Pascal wrote: 'All of humanity's problems stem from man's inability to sit quietly in a room alone.' Dallas Willard writes about solitude: 'Solitude well practised will break the power of busyness, haste, isolation and loneliness. You will see that the world is not on your shoulders after all. You will find yourself and God will find you in new ways' (Willard, *The Great Omission*).

Although solitude can be incredibly uncomfortable – especially for those of us who are extroverts – as we embrace it as vocation, in expectation that God will be at work in and through it, we may find, as Henri Nouwen did, that 'Solitude is the furnace of transformation' (Nouwen, *The Way of the Heart*).

As well as making peace with long hours by ourselves during serious illness, we may also need to invite people to accompany us as we journey through dark and fearful places. Yet any who have faced their own times of darkness will know the challenge of finding wise companions who are willing to accompany us in the dark. It can be hard to know whom to trust, and who has the courage to offer accompaniment as we name our darkest fears. We can be surrounded by a community of love and support, but sometimes people's own discomfort leads them to want to rescue us rather than accompany us. Phrases like, 'But you mustn't think like that' imply that naming the darkness isn't allowed, and the constant reminder about the benefits of 'a positive attitude' can compel us to hide our inner darkness from ourselves and others.

In her book, *Learning to Walk in the Dark*, Barbara Brown Taylor notices that difficult and dark emotions are often shut down and suppressed within our contemporary culture:

> Emotions such as grief, fear and despair have gained a reputation as 'the dark emotions' not because they are noxious or abnormal but because Western culture keeps them shuttered in the dark with other shameful things like personal bankruptcy or sexual deviance. If you have ever spent time in the company of dark emotions, you too may have received subtle messages from friends and strangers alike that you were supposed to handle them and move on sooner instead of later. (p. 77)

Taking time to allow ourselves to face the dark emotions during a journey of suffering isn't always easy. It is tempting to avoid naming and acknowledging the deepest moments of desolation, and it can be hard to allow tears to flow because we fear that if we begin to let them out then they might never stop. Articulating these moments of despair to sensitive friends and prayerful supporters is often the first step in allowing ourselves to feel the feelings that are so daunting to acknowledge. When supporting a person going through an experience of darkness, there may be nothing useful to say, and attempts at explanations may only increase the sense of isolation, but quiet accompaniment can be such a blessing. These people will be able to hold the Christ-light for us, while also being our companions in the dark.

Jesus chooses to go out from the Passover meal with his disciples to a quiet place, the garden of Gethsemane, and having gone there, Jesus 'began to be deeply distressed and troubled' (Mark 14.33). It is night, and so the physical darkness mirrors the spiritual darkness in Jesus' soul. John Mark Comer suggests that Jesus chose to go to this quiet garden because he knew that by taking some time in quiet, away from the noise and bustle of Jerusalem at Passover, he would be compelled to confront the raw and intense emotions about what lay ahead of him. Jesus could have chosen not to think about it, but instead he gave himself time to feel the dark feelings of all that he was facing, and then to bring them to God in prayer (Comer, 'Gethsemane Prayer').

Jesus invites just a couple of the disciples to accompany him in his deep distress: 'He took Peter and the two sons of Zebedee along with him, and he began to be sorrowful and troubled. Then he said to them: "My soul is overwhelmed with sorrow to the point of death. Stay here and keep watch with me"' (Matthew 26.37–38).

Jesus needed trusted companions to help him to carry the emotional burden of the cross as he contemplated all that it would mean. Having gathered a community around him in so many different ways within the Gospel stories, here we see Jesus needing emotional support as he faces his own time of profound darkness. In this moment, he didn't need his companions' advice; he needed their attentive presence and prayer.

One of my favourite children's books is *The Owl who was Afraid of the Dark* by Jill Tomlinson, which I enjoyed using during a previous vocation as a primary-school teacher. It tells the story of Plop, a baby barn owl, whose mum sends him out each night to explore some of the gifts of the darkness, in order that he might no longer be so scared of it. Through seven chapters, Plop meets various interesting people and discovers that dark can be exciting, kind, fun, necessary, fascinating, wonderful and beautiful. As I faced my own fear of the dark during the long months of chemotherapy, God sent me a noisy tawny owl one night, hooting outside my window, making sure I heard him, and reassuring me that he wasn't afraid of the dark. This owl returned to keep me company on other occasions, and became a symbol for me of God's loving care, even during my own darkest night.

George Matheson was a Scottish minister in the nineteenth century, who wrote the beautiful hymn 'O love, that wilt not let me go' with its poignant reminder that in times when we feel unable to hold on to God, God still holds on to us. Matheson had been engaged, but his fiancée ended the relationship when he began to lose his sight, saying 'I do not want to be the wife of a blind man.' Years later, having been reminded of that deeply painful moment, he wrote:

> My hymn was composed in the manse of Innellan on the evening of the 6th of June, 1882, when I was 40 years of age. I was alone in the manse at that time. It was the night of my sister's marriage, and the rest of the family were staying overnight in Glasgow. Something happened to me, which was known only to myself, and which caused me the most severe mental suffering.
>
> The hymn was the fruit of that suffering. It was the quickest bit of work I ever did in my life. I had the impression of having it dictated to me by some inward voice rather than of working it out myself. I am quite sure that the whole work was completed in five minutes, and equally sure that it never received at my hands any retouching or correction.

As Matheson faced the reality of the physical darkness of his blindness, so he faced the emotional darkness of being abandoned by his fiancée, and then the further loneliness of his sister preparing to get married. The hymn that the Spirit inspired him to write that evening is extraordinary for its honesty about Matheson's pain, as well as its tender hope in God's redeeming presence. I listened to this hymn again and again during my darkest days, finding it a source of deep comfort and hope.

O love that wilt not let me go,
I rest my weary soul in thee;
I give thee back the life I owe,
That in thine ocean depths its flow
May richer, fuller be.

O Light that follows all my way,
I yield my flick'ring torch to thee;
My heart restores its borrowed ray,
That in thy sunshine's blaze its day
May brighter, fairer be.

O Joy that seekest me thru' pain,
I cannot close my heart to thee;
I trace the rainbow thru' the rain
And feel the promise is not vain
That morn shall tearless be.

O cross that liftest up my head,
I dare not ask to fly from thee;
I lay in dust life's glory dead,
And from the ground there blossoms red
Life that shall endless be.

4

Called to vulnerability

A couple of weeks after my final dose of chemotherapy, I was invited to have my assessment scan in preparation for the radiotherapy. This was at a different hospital, which brought with it additional worries about parking and traffic and finding the right treatment room, as well as the usual unknowns about what would happen at the scan. Eventually a nurse called my name, offered me a hospital gown, and directed me towards a changing room where I could put it on. Emerging from the changing room, I felt cold and embarrassed in the thin gown, with my lopsided silhouette after my mastectomy. I was told to wait in the corridor until my name was called, and other patients and staff walked past and looked at me sympathetically. I felt really vulnerable, and it was a reminder that vulnerability takes many different forms during a cancer journey.

Western society places profound value on human autonomy and choice, and in our ability to make our own decisions about relationships, work, homes and hobbies. As we make our way through our childhood and teenage years, initiative and independence are celebrated as a healthy part of preparing for adulthood, when our journey into autonomy reaches its climax.

In contrast, as soon as a serious illness becomes part of our life, we are propelled into a place of extreme vulnerability. We find ourselves in the hands of doctors, nurses and medical systems, having to trust people that we barely know with one of our most valuable assets – our health. We trust anaesthetists and surgeons to bring their 'A game' to our care, and not to be having a bad day. We trust the advice of our medical teams, amidst the vulnerability of recognizing that some aspects of treatment aren't an exact science, and we could plausibly get different advice from a different medic on a different day. Suddenly 'clerical errors' aren't just annoying, they take on the weight of life and death, and everything has a greater sense of anxious urgency and pressure.

As the person in the midst of this whirlwind of medical systems and procedures, we take on the status and vocation of a 'patient'. No longer are we invited to define ourselves by our career trajectory, social network, education and family. We are now defined by a hospital number, a diagnosis and a treatment plan. No longer are we free to make our own choices and manage our own schedules. We now need to put ourselves in the hands of surgeons, anaesthetists, oncologists, nurses and radiographers, and allow them to direct our journey.

Entering into this place of profound vulnerability can be immensely uncomfortable, and this vulnerability extends right through the treatment and beyond. There is vulnerability in waiting for the diagnosis and treatment plan, and then in waiting to see if the treatment has been successful. There is vulnerability in showing to numerous medics parts of our bodies that would usually remain hidden, and revealing our nakedness to those who approach it as scientists rather than lovers. There is vulnerability in sitting in corridors wearing hospital gowns or attached to drips, looking and feeling profoundly unwell while in a public place.

In response to this sense of vulnerability, numerous books about cancer focus on reclaiming autonomy, using phrases like, 'Take control of your cancer', 'Take back your life from cancer', 'Become the boss of your cancer'. Though these sentiments can be helpful in stirring courage and confidence, there is also much to learn from the experience of, and vocation to, vulnerability. Because, just as our vulnerability compels us to place ourselves in the hands of medics, so we can once again place ourselves in the even firmer hands of our loving and ever-present God.

The Stature of Waiting, by W. H. Vanstone, is a concise exploration of the significance of Jesus' vulnerability and what it means for humanity. Drawing on the Greek word '*pascho*', from which we get the English word 'passion', Vanstone points out that the most direct translation of this word is 'to be done unto', and that 'at a certain point in His life, Jesus passed from action to passion, from the role of subject to that of object and from working in freedom to waiting upon what others decided and receiving what others did' (p. 31).

Vanstone goes on to argue that we see something of the nature and glory of God when Jesus becomes vulnerable, is 'handed over', and becomes the one who is done unto, rather than the agent of the action. God is therefore not only recognized in power and strength, but also in the ways that Jesus chooses the path of weakness and vulnerability.

The English word 'patient' takes its origin, via Latin, from the same Greek word, '*pascho*'. Vanstone writes movingly about the moment when someone's identity becomes primarily that of a patient:

> To a person who, in the prime of life, is suddenly struck down by a serious accident or by a debilitating disease ... there often comes a moment when he recognizes his helplessness ... Thereupon his place and status in the world undergoes a sudden and remarkable change. Up to this point he was ordering and arranging his own affairs and, very probably, the affairs of a number of other people also. He was holding the reins of a team of projects and purposes – major and minor, public and private; he was taking action, initiating policy, making decisions. (p. 34)

This change from active to passive, from strength to vulnerability, from supporting others to relying on others, is a stark and emotional transition to go through. But Vanstone points out that, if we do indeed see the glory of God revealed in Jesus as he goes through his own time of vulnerability, there are implications for how we should view vulnerability ourselves. Understanding ourselves as reflecting the glory of God when we are weak and vulnerable, as well as when we are confident and competent, can challenge and reframe how we relate to our own weakness.

St Paul writes most directly about his own experience of vulnerability in 2 Corinthians 12, when he refers to a 'thorn in my flesh' from which God doesn't heal him (12.7). Instead, he senses God saying to him, 'My grace is sufficient for you, for my power is made perfect in weakness' (12.9). He goes on to declare, 'That is why, for Christ's sake, I delight in weaknesses, in insults, in hardships, in persecutions, in difficulties. For when I am weak, then I am strong' (12.10). This is one of the paradoxes of the Christian faith, that sometimes it is in our weakness and frailty that we are most able to live out our true vocations as creatures before our creator God, and as children of our Heavenly Father.

Making peace with our own limitations and vulnerability is a lifelong journey, but one that can be hastened during a time of illness, when we are forced to face the truth that we are not sovereign over ourselves and our circumstances. In their powerful book, *Jesus Wept*, Vanessa Herrick and Ivan Mann explain:

> In living with ourselves and with other people it is all too easy to try to forget our finitude, to hang onto some illusive and false strength which we like to imagine will save us from the human condition. But it is to the fullness of the human condition that we are called with all its vulnerability, risks, temptations and fears as well as its joys and delights. (p. 63)

Herrick and Mann further give the example of a hospital chaplain who suddenly found herself in the position of patient rather than chaplain. They write:

> She thought at first that she needed to acknowledge that she could no longer minister there. Then she realized that her ministry lay, for now, in being powerless, not powerful, and that in the way she allowed others to minister to her, she might reflect

> Christ's own ministry of handing over to others in surrender to God. (p. 132)

It was halfway through my five months of chemotherapy treatment that I decided that it was time to shave my head. Though I'd kept quite a good amount of hair around my ears, it was significantly thinned on the top, and more and more was falling out every time I brushed it; so I was already wearing a bandana most of the time. The children helped with the shave, and we used the shaver that we, like many other families, had bought during the Covid-19 pandemic when barbers were closed. This was a big moment, and, although I'd been preparing the children for the fact that it would eventually become necessary, it wasn't easy for any of us. This was such a visual sign that I was ill, and that things had changed.

Whether I wore a headscarf or went out bald, it was now very obvious that I had made the transition from confident vicar of a large church to cancer patient, and I felt a deep shyness and vulnerability in going out with my new look. For each outing and each encounter, I needed to muster courage, put on my confident smile, and try to look normal, even though I knew that I now looked very clearly like someone who was having chemotherapy. My identity was now visibly as someone with cancer, and I felt the discomfort deeply.

In these moments of vulnerability, it can be especially hard to go out into the world, and to present ourselves in our suffering. Pete Greig expresses it like this: 'There's something about suffering that makes us want to curl up in a ball and hide our vulnerability because we don't want to expose the soft parts of our lives' (Staton, 'Ask, Seek, Knock').

In my discomfort at my very visible vulnerability, I had a deep sense of the importance of showing it to my church community, however tempting it was to return to my safe cocoon and keep my vulnerability hidden. Though I might prefer to be seen as strong, confident and able, in this season I knew that I was called to be present in my church community as a fellow Christian first, and as a vicar second. Suffering is the great equalizer, and as I allowed the church family to see me and love me in my vulnerability, I sensed that God would do something profound in our midst. Turning up at church wearing a headscarf, or with my bald head, became the very visible way of showing my vulnerability, and, although it was initially very uncomfortable, it gradually got easier. Describing his own experience of vulnerability during his cancer treatment, Tyler Staton explained:

> I was losing everything except Christ in front of everyone. I was losing my strength, losing my ability to control my world to much of any degree, losing my looks, eyebrows, eye-lashes falling out, and everything else. I was losing my ability to show up in many of the ways I'd got used to as a pastor ... I had gotten used to showing up to people through my strengths ... Suddenly I was just weak, and all I could offer to people was my weakness. And God taught me things through that that I'm still getting words for. (Staton, 'Lessons from His Cancer Journey')

At the heart of the Christian faith is the concept that we can't save ourselves, that we need the gracious, sacrificial action of God in Jesus to redeem us and restore us, and that we receive that gift when we humbly acknowledge our need of it. Twelve-Step recovery groups, like Alcoholics Anonymous, also begin with a comprehensive and humble expression of need: 'I'm X, and I'm an alcoholic.' Acknowledging this deep vulnerability, and inability to save ourselves, is seen within Twelve-Step communities as a vital and profound moment of surrender, and it is understood that only from that place of powerlessness and vulnerability can true healing begin.

During my sick leave, Bishop Ruth Bushyager covered Holy Week and Easter at St Mary's, and spoke movingly on Maundy Thursday about the importance of vulnerability within Christian communities:

> We think that the gold standard in Christian living is to be a really sorted person, someone who never has mental-health challenges, someone who never has physical ailments, someone who never wrestles with spiritual doubts and someone who's materially successful, because then we can be strong servants of the church, as we give and give to others, out of our own strength and wellness. But if we live like that, we shut the door on every kind of divine goodness.

There is a depth of faith and trust that can grow only when we are vulnerable, when we are taken beyond our own capabilities and strength and invited to rely on God in our weakness. Strahan Coleman explains the significance of that moment in his own experience: 'But then something important happened. I gave up. I gave up on being able to pray, on understanding what was going on with me, on waiting for it all to be fixed and on needing answers' (Coleman, *Beholding*, Chapter 1). There is a spiritual vulnerability in these moments that comes from not having answers to the most profound questions of suffering. By relinquishing our need for everything to be explained, we are enabled to invite God simply to show himself to us in his love.

In the Book of Exodus, God rescues the Israelites from slavery in Egypt, but they are then led into the desert, where they fear that they will die. God promises to provide them with bread (manna) for each morning, and meat (quail) for each evening, but commands them firmly not to take more than they need, and instead to trust God for their daily provision. However, this was very difficult for the Israelites to do. They wanted to take plenty of food and store it up for the days ahead, so that they could be in charge of organizing their provision. But God wanted them to trust him with their hunger, to trust that he would provide enough food for each of them for each day. It's extraordinary to note that this daily provision of manna in the desert lasted for 40 years. For 40 years, the Israelites would wake up hungry each morning with nothing in the cupboard, and step outside with their vulnerability and need, to find the provision that God had miraculously offered for them.

It can be complex to hold together both our competence and our vulnerability and to find ways to integrate these two parts of ourselves. Henri Nouwen wrote *The Inner Voice of Love* as a series of entreaties to himself as he journeyed through a difficult season of disintegration. He writes this:

> There is within you a lamb and a lion. Spiritual maturity is the ability to let lamb and lion lie down together. Your lion is your adult, aggressive self. It is your initiative-taking and decision-making self. But there is also your fearful, vulnerable lamb, the part of you that needs affection, support, affirmation, and nurturing. When you heed only your lion, you will find yourself over-extended and exhausted. When you take notice only of your lamb, you will easily become a victim of your need for other people's attention. The art of spiritual living is to fully claim both your lion and your lamb. Then you can act assertively without denying your own needs. And you can ask for affection and care without betraying your talent to offer leadership. (p. 67)

Vulnerability is part of the nature of God that we see in the life of Jesus, as well as the nature of humanity made in God's image, and it will therefore be a vocation that we will all be called to inhabit in different ways at different times in our lives. Seeing this vulnerability as gift rather than as restriction may enable us to journey through the discomfort and find hope and purpose within it. Reflecting prayerfully on Jesus' vulnerability as he faced the cross may help us to make peace with the seasons when we are particularly called to vulnerability, as well as renewing our trust in the God who holds us through it.

5

Called to community

My husband and I were looking forward to celebrating our fifteenth wedding anniversary in the summer of 2025, but instead my husband spent the summer driving me to my weekly chemotherapy and then supporting me through the difficult side effects. Our marriage vows to love one another, 'for better, for worse ... in sickness and in health', took on a new meaning, and my husband shouldered a heavy burden of responsibility for me and the children through the long months of treatment.

When we are seriously ill, the burden of worry for our close family can be enormous. They are the ones who maintain a prayerful vigil during surgery, and who watch as our body is battered by chemotherapy and other treatments. Watching loved ones suffer and feeling impotent to help can be as painful as being the one going through the treatment, and the emotional strain for family members can be huge. When there are children within the immediate family there is a further complexity in knowing how much to tell them and when, trying to be honest while not worrying them unnecessarily. Moments of holding my children as they sobbed out their fears about what the cancer might mean were some of the hardest moments of the whole journey for me. As I lay in bed during the long five months of chemotherapy, one of my children reflected, 'I miss you, mum. I know you're still here, but I miss you being you.'

For those who are single when facing illness and treatment, there are different challenges. A friend who went through a year of cancer treatment when single in her 30s commented, 'I guess the hardest thing is that the rest of your life doesn't stop and wait for you. Some days you feel rubbish, but the dog still needs walking and the bills still need paying.'

A diagnosis of cancer very quickly has an impact beyond just the patient and their immediate family. Friends, colleagues and church community will also be affected by the news, and often want to help. Managing the complex network of relationships through the illness can be a further complication for the patient, while the community around them may worry about being in touch too much, or not enough, about saying the wrong thing or saying it at the wrong time. Yet being surrounded by community is such a gift during cancer treatment, and there is an opportunity for a church community to be proactive in offering sensitive love and support.

I was taken to three weeks of daily radiotherapy by a rota of people, on which family, friends and church members all took their places. Everyone wanted to help, and I could easily have filled the rota twice over. It involved an hour each way in the car to the hospital, and then waiting with me in the hospital waiting room for up to an hour until I was called in for my 15-minute appointment. It was noticeable that most people were in the waiting room in pairs; we were encouraged not to drive ourselves home from our treatment if at all possible because one of the side effects is significant tiredness. One day, a run-down and stressed-looking man in his 50s joined the busy waiting room on his own. A nurse came to ask him if he'd brought various forms and medications with him, and he looked blankly at her, and then started to cry. Through his tears, he explained that it was hard enough for him to get himself to the hospital on the bus, and that he didn't realize that he was supposed to bring anything with him. The nurse tried to reassure him that she'd sort it out, but he looked so lonely and isolated, and my heart broke for him. I reflected on how hard it must be to face cancer treatment alone, and I was reminded again of how blessed I was to be surrounded by such an extensive and loving community.

The importance of community is modelled for us as Christians when we reflect on the beautiful relationships between the three persons of the Trinity, and the way that they exist in a dance of reciprocity and love. As Christians, made in the image of God, we are made for relationship and community, and invited to join the loving relationships within the Trinity. As the Croation theologian Miraslav Volf writes:

> Because the Christian God is not a lonely God, but rather a communion of three persons, faith leads human beings into the divine communion. One cannot, however, have a self-enclosed communion with the Triune God – a 'foursome', as it were – for the Christian God is not a private deity. Communion with this God is at once also communion with those others who have entrusted themselves in faith to the same God. (Volf, *After our Likeness*)

Being made in the image of God means that all of humanity is made for community, and belonging to communities of various forms is part of our universal vocation. As Christians, we share a further vocation to community within 'the body of Christ', which is Paul's foundational image for the church in the New Testament (for example, 1 Corinthians 12.12–27 and Ephesians 1.22–23). Whether we meet with our Christian family on a Sunday or within a midweek home group, whether the meetings are daily, weekly or monthly, in person or online, being a Christian means that we belong to one another as the body of Christ, within the worldwide church, as well as within our local congregations and communities of believers. These Christian communities are never perfect, and finding our places within them can often be complex and always changing. Yet they are the communities where we learn to love and to be loved, and where we are reminded that we aren't just a social club of like-minded people: we are the body of Christ, and we belong to one another as well as to God.

Jesus also needed community around him during his earthly vocation, calling twelve disciples to be his close companions, as well as sharing deep friendships with the siblings Mary, Martha and Lazarus. In our society where self-sufficiency is seen as a goal, and if not self-sufficiency then balanced reciprocity, it's not easy to receive kindness from others with no strings attached. Bishop Ruth Bushyager also explored this theme within her Maundy Thursday sermon in Horsham:

> As an adult, we never see self-sufficiency in Jesus. He depends on his Heavenly father and all kinds of people to meet his basic needs ... receiving baptism from his cousin; receiving dinner from Zacchaeaus; receiving shelter and food from Martha and Mary. He borrows someone else's boat and someone else's donkey; receives water from a cup given from a Samaritan woman ... He receives wine vinegar from Roman soldiers. He receives burial in someone else's tomb. The Lord of the Universe lives in a way that makes him indebted to the community around him.

Communities within work, leisure and church that we used to belong to and relate to easily may not be so easy to access when we are receiving treatment, and yet finding nurturing and supportive communities is so vital in sustaining our emotional and spiritual well-being. During treatment, my immediate community of daily and weekly contacts became much smaller, and often I really wanted to hear stories of other people's lives and what was going on for them. As I began to explain this to my friends, several of them started sending me regular WhatsApp messages with their news, which helped me to feel connected when my social contact had shrunk. My weekly netball club became one of the highlights of my week; a female community where I was 'Lisa' rather than 'the vicar' and where I could maintain some kind of normality while also receiving gentle and loving support. I attended as often as I could, always playing a netball position that didn't involve too much running. They were also the first community that I felt brave enough to show my bald head to – it wasn't easy wearing a headscarf on the netball court.

Relating to our Christian community can also feel harder during illness, when the normal patterns of worship and fellowship are no longer accessible because of reduced immunity or physical limitations. I felt the impact of this change particularly as a Christian minister, no longer able to offer the pastoral leadership and ministry that I had been called to. But it's not just clergy who can find the transition difficult. Whether our church vocations have been as a welcomer, helping with the children's work, or doing pastoral visiting, it can be uncomfortable to find ourselves no longer able to offer the gifts to the church community that we have valued. We may now find that we need others to minister to us, rather than being the ones who do the giving ourselves. We may find ourselves marginalized within the Christian communities in which we had previously been central.

Serious illness can be a very lonely time, not least because of the sense that no one will really understand the unique circumstances and challenges that illness has forced upon us. As the psychologist Carl Jung expressed it: 'Loneliness doesn't come from being alone, but from being unable to communicate the things that seem important to you' (Jung, *Memories, Dreams, Reflections*). It can also be a challenge to find words to express how we're feeling, and that makes it even harder to reach out, as Strahan Coleman explains:

> Though it didn't help one bit, I tried my best to hide the depths of both my physical struggle and my emotional struggle from those around me. I couldn't explain it to them, so I hardly tried. (Coleman, *Beholding*, Chapter 1)

In the early days of my diagnosis, I didn't really want to see anyone apart from my close family. I was grateful to be in touch with friends on WhatsApp, and I sent emails to update the church community about how my treatment was going, but I wasn't ready for visits. I didn't have words for how I felt, apart from a pervading sense of numbness. I valued quiet time with my husband and children, doing jigsaws, watching easy TV, and allowing my mind to process all that was happening. As the weeks went by, I began to invite a few trusted friends and colleagues to visit, and gradually I became more confident in seeing the church family and wider community around me. By Easter Sunday, four months after being signed off from work and halfway through my chemotherapy, I was ready to stand at the church door and offer Easter greetings to the 500 worshippers. I valued different things at each stage of the journey, from needing a significant time of hibernation following my diagnosis, to gradually feeling able to reach out to the individuals and communities who were holding me in their love and prayers.

Many people have cancer stories to share, and everyone's story is different. There can be moments when others want to share their story with you but you don't really want to hear it! Then at other moments, hearing of others' experiences can ease the sense of loneliness and resonate deeply with your own journey. My husband valued coffee-chats through the cancer journey with a dad-friend who had had his own cancer experience as a young man – our children were in the same class. It meant a lot to our children that this dad had also had cancer and come through it.

I received up-to-date breast-cancer advice from a lovely parishioner, Sarah, a similar age to me, who was a year through her breast-cancer treatment, and had already experienced chemotherapy, surgery and radiotherapy. Her warm manner and positivity were such a gift in the early days, and I always remember her saying that she treated each test and procedure as the scientist that she was, seeing them as a fascinating opportunity to learn how these things worked. I liked this approach, and so I endeavoured to embark on my MRI, bone scan, heart-function test, biopsies and other treatments with that sense of intrigue and opportunity to learn.

In my previous career as a teacher, if I'd been diagnosed with serious cancer, I'd probably have been signed off work for many months and may not have seen anyone from work during that period. However, as a vicar, I had been called to an incarnational ministry, living within the community where I served. For me, that meant living 100 metres away from our large and busy church, on a beautiful and historic road, popular with tourists and locals. Being a vicar isn't a nine-to-five job that can be left behind at the end of the day to return home. It is a whole-life vocation, and I had been called to share my life with my congregation in a particular way. However, that didn't mean that there weren't boundaries, and it didn't mean that I needed to share everything. Just as my congregation valued their own privacy, they were so loving in the ways that they understood and respected my need for privacy during my treatment.

The complication was that I couldn't go out of my front door without bumping into several parishioners and members of the local community, and so I quickly learnt that if I wanted to go out, I needed to feel ready for a conversation, and to have answers prepared. When they asked the inevitable, 'How are you?' I tended to offer a quick summary of where I'd got to with the treatment: 'Seven chemo doses done now, nine more to go.' And then something more general like, 'It's not easy, but we're so fortunate to be surrounded by so much support.' A clergy friend facing a similar cancer journey reflected on how hard it was when many of her congregation said to her 'You're looking so well,' even though she was in pain and she knew that the cancer was growing. She learnt to say, 'Well, appearances can be deceptive, but I'm doing OK at the moment, thank you.'

These conversations and encounters can come to feel uncomfortably formulaic, and yet this approach is often necessary. People are asking because they genuinely care, because they are praying for us and are pleased to see us. They want to know how we are doing, and we want to give them something honest from our encounter. But for a public figure, it can be complicated when there are so many people to communicate with, and it becomes hard to choose how much to share and which bits.

The Christian comedian Steve Legg was interviewed for a podcast in 2024, a few months before his death from cancer (Legg et al., 'Where is God?'). He talked about going to *New Wine*, the large Christian summer conference, where his high profile meant that wherever he went, people would ask him how he was, and they didn't always take the hint when he said, 'Fine' and tried to walk away. A harder aspect of being surrounded by such a loving and praying community is that it's not always easy to have normal conversations on the days when you don't want to talk about the cancer. One of my children expressed a similar view: 'I don't want everyone always asking me about my mum. I don't want to be the child whose mum has got cancer. I just want to be normal.'

We can be surrounded by offers of help and care, but it's not easy to take up the offers, and we may fear becoming a burden, or asking for help from those who are already overwhelmed by their own pressures. Yet, as we grow in confidence in sharing something of our experiences and of our fear and pain, it can lead to healthy and helpful connection with others, as we share something of our burdens and allow them to offer both sympathy and empathy.

Tyler Staton's wife arranged for church members to read to him during the long hours when he received chemotherapy. They would read out loud to him for up to five hours at a time, often reading the Psalms and some of the spiritual classics. Staton reflects that he was too weak to reciprocate; so he just received and received. It came to feel for him that these church members had been like Jesus, ministering the love of God to him, and he noticed that no one else on the cancer ward was receiving the same deep and sacrificial generosity.

In our parish, in response to the overwhelming number of people saying, 'Please tell us how we can help', we asked the church community to provide weekly meals for our family. We also regularly received cards, flowers and gifts on the vicarage doorstep. These gestures were a precious reminder that we were being held in the love and prayers of our church family through the treatment. Luke's Gospel includes the story of some men bringing a paralytic to Jesus, carried on a mat (Luke 5.17–26). When they are prevented by the crowds from reaching Jesus, they make a hole in the roof instead and lower the man down.

It's a story of deep care for the paralysed man, and tenacity on the part of his friends, and I sensed that the persistent prayers of the church community were bringing me before Jesus with the same tenacious love.

Our church had been very involved in welcoming Ukrainians to Horsham following Russia's invasion in 2022, and we were also able to welcome a lovely mother and her teenage daughter from Kyiv into our spacious vicarage. During the hardest days of chemotherapy, our Ukrainian guests made me borscht each week: a wonderful Ukrainian soup, full of healthy ingredients. When the wider Horsham Ukrainian community heard about my cancer, they clubbed together to give us several generous gift tokens for family meals out. It felt humbling to receive such generosity from these Ukrainians who had themselves been through so much.

As we join the communities of those who are being treated for cancer, relationships can be formed quickly and easily by our shared experiences. There's a beautiful sense of taking our place in a stream of cancer-experienced folk, learning from the wisdom of those who've gone before us, and then supporting those who come after us. On my chemotherapy days, I'd often have the opportunity to chat to other women who'd finished their chemotherapy and were back for six-monthly transfusions to reduce the chance of recurrence. I could often tell how long ago their chemotherapy had been by how much their hair had re-grown!

Finding creative ways to access community during treatment, reminding ourselves that we are made for community and reaching out with honesty about what we need may come to be a blessing for us and for those who love us and support us. The first step is having the courage to reach out, as Charlie Mackesy illustrates so clearly in his beautiful book, *The Boy, the Mole, the Fox and the Horse*:

> 'What's the bravest thing you've ever said?' asked the boy.
> 'Help,' said the horse.

6

An embodied calling

When we are diagnosed with a serious physical illness, there can be a sense that our body has let us down. Most of us take our physical health for granted and don't really think about the complexities of how our bodies work, until suddenly there is a problem, and scary words like 'cancer' come to form part of our story and experience. The physical scars of surgery can leave us feeling mutilated and deformed, reluctant to look at ourselves in the mirror when it reminds us of all that we've been through.

We are likely to find ourselves regularly hearing the refrain, 'You need to listen to your body', but intense treatments like chemotherapy can leave us feeling that we don't recognize our bodies and our physical reactions any longer. I found it especially frustrating when my mind was ready to return to work, ready for contact and life again, but my body was going gradually downhill, as the cumulative effects of the chemotherapy started to be felt. Later on, I noticed that I was well enough to feel bored, but not yet well enough to return to work, and that also felt complicated. As we journey through different stages of treatment, over days, weeks, months and years, it's not easy to listen tenderly to what our body might be telling us, or to respond to it with care and patience.

We may need to grieve for the ways that our bodies have let us down. It may take time to befriend again our physical frame, and to make peace with its new shape and limitations. Grieving all that we've gone through can itself be a very physical process, as the novelist Liane Moriarty expresses:

> It felt like her parents were sick with a terrible, incurable disease that ravaged their bodies. It felt like they'd been assaulted. As if someone had come after them with a baseball bat. She had not realized that grief was so physical. Before Zach died, she thought grief happened in your head. She didn't know that your whole body ached with it, that it screwed up your digestive system, your menstrual cycle, your sleep patterns, your skin. (Moriarty, *Nine Perfect Strangers*, p. 205)

Being reminded that God made and loves our physical bodies may help us to treat ourselves tenderly, and to continue to respect and honour our physicality, even in its weakness. Joni Eareckson Tada, who became a quadriplegic following a diving accident when she was just 17, writes:

> When I get up in the morning – as difficult as it is – I need to remember in whose image I am made. My body may be broken, but I am a God-reflector. I mirror a God who made me in his image. And that is what gives me (gives us all) human dignity – not the ability to walk or use of your hands. (Eareckson Tada, 'We Are Image-Bearers of God')

On a post-surgery visit with my surgeon, himself a Christian, he commented about the human body, 'It's the most extraordinary design.' It was particularly moving to hear a surgeon reflecting on the miraculous complexity of the human body, and the way that God had created it. It reminded me of the words of Psalm 139: 'I praise you because I am fearfully and wonderfully made' (139.14).

Christianity has always affirmed the value and significance of the material world and our physical bodies, with Archbishop William Temple calling Christianity 'the most avowedly materialistic of all religions' (*Nature, Man and God*, p. 478). Genesis, Chapter 1, teaches that humanity has been given the profound dignity of being made in the image of God (Genesis 1.26) and further that God looked at all that he had created and 'saw that it was very good' (Genesis 1.31). In the incarnation, the early Christians came to understand that Jesus Christ was both fully God and fully human, 'For in Christ all the fullness of the Deity lives in bodily form' (Colossians 2.9). During his ministry, Jesus frequently used physical touch when offering healing (Luke 4.40), as well as using earthly things like mud and spit (John 9.6–7).

In his resurrection appearances, Jesus' body was still physical, and, although it clearly had some unique differences (he could travel through walls to enter into a locked room – John 20.19), he was still able to eat fish with the disciples (Luke 24.42–43) and encouraged Thomas to reach out to him physically: 'Put your finger here; see my hands. Reach out your hand and put it into my side. Stop doubting and believe' (John 20.27).

There was pressure from the ideas of Gnosticism in the first and second centuries, influenced by Platonic philosophy, to consider that only spiritual things were good, and to view the physical aspects of existence with suspicion and distrust. However, the early Christians continued to argue that the goodness of God could be found in physical things, and to use water, bread and wine within the sacramental life of the church. Responding to the thought of Pope John Paul II on this subject, the Catholic theologian Christopher West wrote, 'The theology of the body is a clarion call for the Church not to become more "spiritual", but to become more incarnational. It is a call to allow the Word of the Gospel to penetrate our flesh and bones' (West, 'Theology of the Body').

The value that Christianity places on our physical bodies means that they also play an important part in our life of faith and our vocation, as St Paul writes to the Corinthians: 'Do you not know that your bodies are temples of the Holy Spirit, who is in you, whom you have received from God? You are not your own, you were bought at a price. Therefore honour God with your body' (1 Corinthians 6.19–20). It's easy to minimize quite how significant this idea was for the earliest Christians in the aftermath of Pentecost: that the Holy Spirit of God had come to dwell within the bodies of Christians. Yet even in the light of the foundational

Christian doctrines of the incarnation, and the indwelling Holy Spirit, Strahan Coleman reflects on how Christians have often been at risk of minimizing the role of our bodies in our lives of faith: 'We've bought into enlightenment thinking that the body is just the machine that hosts the real stuff, the conscious self, and isn't a meaningful participant in our communion with God' (Coleman, *Beholding*, Chapter 11).

In British society, the assisted-dying bill has brought us to a time of intense debate around how we treat our physical bodies. Among the complex arguments around assisted dying, those against it express concerns about the negative message it would send to the elderly, seriously ill and disabled, whose physical bodies are weak and tired. Alongside these discussions about how we treat our bodies in our final days and weeks, there has been a very rapid rise in the number of those opting for a direct cremation: 3% in 2019 has risen to 20% in 2023 (Sunlife Cost of Dying Report). A direct cremation, Ysenda Maxtone Graham writes in the *Church Times*, means: 'no ceremony; no one attending; body taken straight to centralized crematorium to be incinerated; family doesn't even know when it's happening; ashes returned by courier within 14 days' (Graham, 'Notebook').

Advertisements for these direct cremations focus on easing the pressure for our loved ones after we've died, and paint idealized visions of all the other things that the money could be spent on instead of a funeral. But direct cremations don't acknowledge the significance of funerals as important rites of passage for the living as well as for the dead. They also minimize the importance of saying goodbye to the person's physical body, which is the way that they've been known and recognized through their lives. As Anne Richards puts it on the Modern Church blog:

> the last acts of love a person can perform for a loved one have always had significance ... Direct cremation interrupts both this sacred understanding of the dead body and the sense that it has deep and powerful spiritual value. Whether offered overtly or not, such a no-fuss service undermines the sense that a dead

> body is worthy of respect, care, dignity and love. (Richards, 'The Death of Us')

As Christians, honouring our physical bodies even when they are frail, even when they let us down, will send a message to a society that increasingly doesn't value our physicality unless it is strong and healthy.

The vocation of St Ignatius of Loyola developed from a time of serious physical limitation and so reminds us of all that God can do in us and through us, even on our sick beds. Ignatius' right leg was shattered in battle by a cannon ball, and he was forced into a long convalescence, during which he was bedridden. He asked for books to read about triumphs in battle but had to settle for biographies of the saints. In his long convalescence he had plenty of time for daydreaming, and sometimes he would dream of great victories and winning the approval of the people at court. At other times, inspired by the stories of the saints, he would daydream about doing great things for God. Gradually Ignatius began to notice that, although he enjoyed both daydreams, the after-effect of the two daydreams was very different. When he dreamed about glory through worldly battles, he was left feeling empty and discontented. But when he dreamed about doing great things for God, he felt a deep peace and contentment afterwards.

From this experience, St Ignatius developed his ideas about the 'discernment of spirits', where one grows in awareness of the things that draw us towards God (bringing consolation) and the things that lead us away from God (bringing desolation). We may be facing a significant challenge, such as a cancer diagnosis, and yet be aware of being drawn towards God through it. Alternatively, we may be busy having fun and doing lots of apparently good things, and yet be aware that, at a deeper level, all is not as it might be, and we are being drawn away from God. When he recovered, Ignatius chose to reject all the trappings of his previous life as a courtier, put on the rough cloth of a pilgrim, and undertake an intense time of prayer and self-examination. His example invites us to trust in the work that God can do in our lives when we are physically incapacitated, if we offer all of ourselves to him, including our struggling bodies.

In Genesis, Chapter 32, we find Jacob under intense pressure, fearful that his brother, Esau, is coming with armies to fight him. In verse 24, Jacob is alone at night with his anxious thoughts, and we're told that 'a man wrestled with him until daybreak.' A few verses later, it emerges that it was God with whom he'd been wrestling, and Jacob is given the name 'Israel' because he has 'struggled with God and with men' and has overcome (v. 28). From this wrestling with God, Jacob's hip is wrenched out of place, so that he walks with a limp (v. 31). Jacob's wound becomes a mark of his deep wrestling with God, and through the discomfort, it becomes a physical reminder of God's presence in his life, and of the moment when he 'saw God face to face' (v. 30).

A friend who recently had bowel cancer introduced me to a song called 'Scars', which was released in 2018 by the American group 'I am They'. This includes the provocative refrain, 'I'm thankful for the scars'. In this profound song, the group explain that they have come to see their scars as a gift because the scars have brought them closer to God, and 'the wounds are a story' that God will use. Just like Jacob's experience, the song invites us to consider that we might be able to see our physical scars differently, as marks of God's work in our lives, because in our brokenness we've been drawn closer to God. Extending the image from Isaiah 53.5, 'By his wounds we are healed', the song continues by speaking of Jesus' scars, and the way that they have brought humanity closer to God. This poignant parallel between our scars and Jesus' scars can become a powerful image to hold onto. As we gaze on Jesus' broken body on the cross, broken for us, we might feel able to offer our own broken bodies too, and allow both to be reminders for us of God's redeeming love and grace and the hope of resurrection. As David Runcorn writes: 'Jesus' resurrection, revealed and recognized by his glorious scars, is the pledge of our transfiguring too – wounds and all' (Runcorn, 'Reflections on the Resurrection').

When he faced his own extended period of serious illness, Strahan Coleman was brought to an unexpected moment of recognizing the role of his physical body in prayer, in being able to express what was needed when his mind couldn't find the words:

> Even though I was unable to consciously commune with God due to the mental exhaustion and fatigue, my body was crying out, interceding for me on my behalf, and it was. I realized that God was more than able to see the pain and struggle of my body, laid out before him, crying out for healing and redemption. (Coleman, *Beholding*, Chapter 11)

What we do with our bodies can be as much a form of prayer as what we do with our minds. In the Old Testament, and particularly the Psalms, there are seven different Hebrew words that are commonly translated as 'praise', but whose literal meaning is much more physical, inviting us to use our whole bodies in worship and prayer. Two of these specifically relate to how we use our hands.

The Hebrew word *yadah* ('We will praise [*yadah*] your name forever'; Psalm 44.8) comes from two root words: *yad*, which means the open hand, direction, power. And *ah*, which refers to Jehovah. Together they literally mean to worship with an extended hand or to lift hands in praise.

Towdah ('I will present my thank-offerings *[towdah]* to you'; Psalm 56.12) comes from the same root as *yadah*, but this time the open hand is in a receiving posture, opening our hands in trust and surrender as we look up to God, aligning ourselves with his will.

Lying on our sick beds, in hospital or at home, we can allow the position of our hands to symbolize our *yadah and towdah* prayer. By raising our hands to God in praise and thanksgiving and opening our hands to God in surrender and trust, we can allow our bodies to pray in moments when we may struggle to find words.

Tears may also become the way that our body prays: a model of prayer that is common in the Bible but which has drifted out of our Christian traditions. At the beginning of 1 Samuel, we see Hannah weeping in the Temple, pouring out her tears before God because she feels that her body has let her down – she is barren. In John 11, we're told that Jesus wept, in grief at the death of Lazarus, and in empathy with the grief of Lazarus' sisters. Psalm 56 contains the beautiful assurance that God sees and counts all our tears: 'You have kept count of my tossings; put my tears in your bottle' (Psalm 56.8, ESV). Allowing tears to become part of our prayer may also enable us to bring our deepest and most pained experiences to God, as Runcorn's book, *The Language of Tears*, beautifully explains:

> Simply because they are a language that has been flowing out of the earliest and most evocative depths of our lives, our relationship to our tears will be complex, mysterious and elusive. A language deeper than words is being expressed here. Through tears our bodies are expressing what is in our hearts. (pp. 8–9)

As I made my way through my treatment, one Sunday I found the words of one of the Anglican prayers after communion taking on a renewed significance: 'we offer you our souls and bodies to be a living sacrifice.' Though our bodies may feel battered and frail and we may not like them very much, perhaps this makes the offering of them to God even more profound. Offering ourselves to God through our debilitating treatment and its consequences means offering to God our tired, broken bodies, knowing that God will receive and honour the offering.

7

Called to be ready to die

I was meeting with a nurse to prepare for having chemotherapy, and her computer screen with my details on it had various sub-pages. As I scanned the headings, my eyes landed on the final one: mortality. Of course, that would be the end of this part of my journey, whether I died from cancer or not, but seeing it on the file with my name on it was stark.

St Benedict challenged his monks to: 'Keep death always before your eyes' (*Rule of St Benedict* 4.47), and, through the centuries, many Christians came to adopt the tradition of having a skull on their desk as a reminder of their mortality. Most of us prefer not to think about our own death until circumstances force us to do so; death is one of the greatest certainties in life, and yet so little time is spent in preparing for it. When death is so hidden within our society, it can increase our fear of it; we even avoid the language of dying, preferring to talk about people having 'passed away'. Yet having a healthy awareness of the reality of death can give us a greater wisdom as we navigate the choices in this life, as Steve Jobs, a founder and former CEO of Apple, explains:

> Remembering that I'll be dead soon is the most important tool I've found for helping me make the big decisions in life. Because almost everything, all external expectations, all pride, all fear of failure, these things just fall away in the face of death. And what is left is what's truly important. (Jobs, 'Stanford Commencement Speech')

As I journeyed with others who were on a similar cancer journey to my own, I became aware that many people are very scared to die. One encounter particularly impacted me, with a remarkable lady who had been a pioneer in her working life. Her cancer had become metastatic and therefore could be managed but not cured. As we chatted, her anxiety was palpable, as she spoke about her fight to stay alive and her fear of needing to be transferred to hospice care.

Society's rhetoric around death is all about fighting to live: that's what people are commended and celebrated for. But it's possible to fight to live at the same time as preparing to die; the two things aren't mutually exclusive. On the chemotherapy ward, there was often a shared spirit of 'we're fighting cancer together', and yet there were moments with very ill patients when I felt the Spirit prompting me to say to them, 'If you want to talk about dying, I don't mind having that conversation with you. Talking about dying doesn't mean that you're going to stop fighting to live.'

When we first talked to the children about my cancer, and they asked the inevitable question, 'Are you going to die?', I had an immediate response for them when I was first diagnosed: 'No. This cancer is treatable, I'm not going to die.' As the weeks and months went on, I found myself responding slightly differently. So when questions about dying came up again, I said instead: 'Yes, definitely, I'm going to die one day, we all are. Probably not for quite a while, but I'm definitely going to die sometime, and then I'll be with God, and it'll be OK.' Framing death differently in conversation with the children felt really important; a way of helping them to prepare for the reality of my death, as well as being able to talk about death itself.

Spending time on a chemotherapy ward also raises the question of who is talking to seriously ill patients about dying. As a vicar, I've often had the privilege of having these frank conversations with parishioners who wanted to plan their funeral, or who wanted to talk about death as they processed a terminal diagnosis. But ever fewer people are part of faith communities, and chaplaincy teams in hospitals are increasingly limited. In conversations with oncologists and with other patients, it became clear that these difficult conversations about dying are just as likely to be avoided on the cancer wards as they are in the rest of society.

Against the backdrop of society's deep-rooted fear of dying and reluctance to talk about it, it becomes even more important that Christians model a different way. This will mean facing honestly the inevitable fears and sense of grief at what will be left behind, but also growing our vision of heaven, and the joy that awaits us there. A clergy friend with terminal cancer sensed that her oncologist was reluctant to talk about dying, and so when they met she said to her directly, 'I'm a Christian, and a vicar; so, although I'm sad about leaving my loved ones, I'm not scared to die. So please tell me honestly, best-case and worst-case scenarios.'

I was reminded of a man that I'd got to know during my curacy, who reached out to the church when he was diagnosed with terminal cancer. He was desperate to stay alive, and was reaching out to God and to Christians with pleading faith for God to heal him. I especially remember that he sent some money to a TV evangelist in order to be sent a 'healing handkerchief'. I don't know that his life was extended, but I do know that, when he asked me about what might happen when he died, I said that I imagined Jesus reaching out his hand to him and welcoming him through death and into the life of eternity. I was moved to be told by his partner that in his last semi-conscious moments, the dying man reached out his hand, as if he was putting it into the hand of Jesus.

Henri Nouwen addresses the fear of death by reminding us of the death that we have already made as Christians, as we affirm again the baptismal promises of dying to the temptations of 'sin, the world and the devil'. We then enter in the present into the eternal life that Jesus offers, and that will continue beyond our physical death.

> Maybe the death you fear is not simply the death at the end of your present life. Maybe the death at the end of your life won't be so fearful if you can die well now. Yes, the real death – the passage from time into eternity, from the transient beauty of this world to the lasting beauty of the next, from darkness into light – has to be made now. (Nouwen, *The Inner Voice of Love*, p. 89)

Full-immersion baptisms offer a powerful reminder of the death that we undergo when we become followers of Christ. 'We were therefore buried with him through baptism into death in order that, just as Christ was raised from the dead through the glory of the Father, we too may live a new life' (Romans 6.4). Rising up from the water, as Christ rose from the tomb, we begin our new life as followers of Christ: 'if anyone is in Christ, the new creation has come: the old has gone, the new is here!' (2 Corinthians 5.17).

It's challenging to consider what it means to handle a terminal diagnosis in a Christian way, grateful for treatment options, but not needing to fight to stay alive at all costs. This is likely to involve deep reflections on death before we face a serious illness, perhaps meditating on biblical verses like: 'whether we live or die, we belong to the Lord' (Romans 14.8) and 'for me, to live is Christ, and to die is gain' (Philippians 1.21). This approach would be profoundly counter-cultural, and therefore a powerful witness in our society. Bishop Mariann Edgar Budde talked in an interview about a friend with a terminal diagnosis, who said to her, 'Just watch me now. I'm going to die as if everything we say in church is true' (Budde, 'How We Learn to be Brave').

The beautiful words of Psalm 139.16 remind us, 'all the days ordained for me were written in your book before one of them came to be', and encourage us to live peacefully with what we've been given, rather than fight desperately for more. Being at peace with living and dying, as well as recognizing that we're not in control of the timetable, is not at all easy, and this is unlikely to be something that we can manufacture by ourselves. This deep peace will be a gift of grace, something that we can seek and pray for, the 'peace of God that transcends all understanding' as Paul describes it in Philippians 4.7. This peace is also unlikely to be a one-off gift. We may find that just when we think we've received peace in being ready to die, something else will trigger tears or anger, and we'll need to bring ourselves before God again, praying that we might be enabled to live peacefully and well within the parameters of the days that he has given us.

One of the 'gifts' of dying of cancer is that we know we're dying, and so we have time to consider what it might mean to die well. It gives us time to say goodbye to loved ones, to let go of relationships and roles that have mattered to us and intentionally entrust them to God and others. Giving ourselves opportunities for healthy grief can also be so significant in supporting the grief journeys of those around us. A clergy colleague who died of cancer aged just 59, while still serving as vicar of his parish, wrote poignantly, 'We live and minister in public, so perhaps shouldn't be surprised that we're ill and die that way too. People have been enormously kind and I'm having the privilege of hearing my eulogy before my funeral – which is weird but good' (Fr Andrew Perry).

A very special church member called Jane had become a powerful role model for our whole church family, when her cancer became terminal. Though she was honest about her sadness in leaving her husband, parents and adult son, she knew where she was going. She knew that Jesus, who had been her faithful companion through life, would continue to walk with her through her death, and there was a radiance within her, even as she physically weakened. In her final weeks, she embodied St Paul's words in 2 Corinthians 4.16: 'Though outwardly we are wasting away, yet inwardly we are being renewed day by day.'

The inspiring Roman Catholic nun Sr Gemma Simmonds tells the story of facing serious surgery, when a doctor asked her if she wanted to be resuscitated, should it be needed. To the doctor's surprise, she answered firmly, 'Definitely not'. As the doctor looked at her, puzzled, she explained, 'I've had a better offer.' Looking forward to the joy of heaven, which will indeed be a 'better offer', can enable us to cling less tightly to our life today.

The reality of the Communion of Saints always feels especially close in our beautiful church of St Mary's, Horsham, where 800 years of faith and prayer have seeped into the walls. Worshipping in old church buildings can lead us to ponder the lives of Christians who have gone before us – their hopes and fears, their faith and doubt. In reflecting on their lives, we can grow in confidence about the promise of eternal life after we die. Anglican Eucharistic prayers always make intentional reference to the reality of the Communion of Saints and the way that our worship on earth is joined with the worship in heaven. Phrases such as, 'Therefore with angels and archangels and with all the company of heaven' and 'with all who stand before you in earth and heaven, we worship you' are prayed week by week in Anglican churches, but I wonder how often we pause to take them in, or allow ourselves to imagine the extraordinary heavenly reality to which they testify.

Julian of Norwich felt called to become an anchoress and so entered into a solitary hermitage: a small cell attached to a church. As was the tradition for those given this calling, as she entered her cell a requiem mass was sung, as if it were her funeral. The entrance to her cell was then bricked up behind her and earth was thrown onto her, as if she was dying and entering her grave. Julian offered such a powerful visual image to the Christians of her day, that in life and in death we belong to God.

Facing a serious health diagnosis, and acknowledging our own mortality, invites us to think deeply about the nature of prayer in times like these. It can be so precious to know that we are surrounded by prayer from our church community, as well as from family and friends. There may be moments when we find ourselves unable to pray, when it becomes even more significant to know that others are praying for us, and holding us before God. We may find ourselves longing that God would do a physical healing within us and asking for people to pray for that healing.

However, we may find ourselves feeling slightly uncomfortable about asking God to perform a miraculous healing for us, when we are aware of others who hadn't received their physical healing, despite the heartfelt prayers of many.

Aware of my public profile within the church and community, I wanted to be careful not to model a faith that is dependent on God giving us what we want or about implying that staying alive is the greatest priority for Christians. I was disturbed to hear another Christian minister, who'd just heard that he was in remission from his serious cancer, saying to his congregation, 'I'm in remission! See, I told you that God is good!' Ministers must be especially careful about this kind of theology, and of making physical healing a proof of God's goodness.

Yet one of the names for God, revealed in Exodus 15.26 (ESV), is 'The Lord, your healer', reminding us that healing is part of the very nature and character of God. Some of us will receive a measure of healing in this life: emotional, spiritual and physical healing. Sometimes this will be through the miracles of modern science and sometimes this will be in ways that science can't explain, and which we may want to attribute directly to our healing God. But any kind of miraculous healing in this life will only be temporary. We will all die eventually. Our ultimate healing will come after death, when we are welcomed into the life of eternity. This will be the moment when all sorrow and suffering will end and 'God will wipe away every tear from their eyes' (Revelation 7.17). As Billy Graham said: 'My home is in heaven. I'm just passing through this world' (Graham, *Just as I am*).

There were moments on the cancer wards, seeing the extraordinary miracle of modern medicine, that I felt profoundly moved by the way that treatments had been developed and were offered to me with skill and care. As I write, in 2025, over 200 different types of cancer have been identified, and are treated by over 100 different types of chemotherapy, as well as immunotherapy, radiotherapy, hormone therapy and bone-marrow transplants (Cancer Research UK). Thousands of doctors and scientists through the years have given their working lives, their energy and their passion to developing and testing models of healing, and we can feel humbled and grateful for their work, and the love of God that has been shown through them.

Tyler Staton reflects on the importance of careful discernment before praying for supernatural healing, and he learnt to ask the question of God: 'How do you want me to pray about this? What should I ask for here?' (Staton, 'Lessons from His Cancer Journey'). Staton's experience of praying this prayer of discernment led him to the point of saying boldly to his church community who were praying for him during his cancer treatment: 'My own discernment and my own prayers, if you want to join them, are for redemption not removal.' Seeing cancer as something that God can redeem, in order to bring good from it, draws on the redemptive model of the cross: the place of despair and desolation that became a place of hope for the world.

Christian healing, as a mark of the kingdom of God, is always about healing in its most holistic sense. Physical healing takes its place alongside emotional healing, spiritual healing, relational healing, community healing and ecological healing, within the wider frame of salvation. Jesus healed the outcast Samaritan woman by spending time with her (John 4), he healed the leper with touch (Matthew 8.3), he healed the unpopular tax-collector by inviting him to become one of his disciples (Matthew 9.9–13). The Greek word used in the Gospels for healing is *sozo*, which can be translated as both healing and salvation. John Mark Comer notices that Jesus seems to intentionally blur the line between the two things, while ancient Christians referred to Jesus as the 'Doctor of the Soul', prompting Comer to point out that salvation is 'not just getting back on the right side of mercy through judicial acquittal but about having your soul healed by God's loving touch' (Comer, *Practising the Way*).

An encounter with our loving God will always bring healing in its most profound and holistic sense. Consequently, when praying for those who are ill, it may be helpful to pray less for specifics related to the nature of the illness, and more that they might encounter God through everything that they're facing. It can be particularly beautiful to pray one of the most simple and ancient prayers of the church: 'Come, Holy Spirit.' This powerful prayer is a prayer of surrender, inviting the Spirit of God to do the beautiful work that she loves to do in our hearts and minds. The Holy Spirit brings perfect healing, not just physical curing in this life, but perfect and eternal healing in body, mind and spirit.

Praying for healing encounters with God for those suffering and their families, for peace and courage to face the harder parts of the journey, and for a vibrant vision of heaven and the joy that awaits us there may be the most appropriate and profound prayer.

8

Called to a new normal

In Charles Dickens' novel *Great Expectations*, we meet the haunted character of Miss Havisham. Jilted at the altar on the day of her wedding, she insists on wearing her wedding dress for the rest of her life, together with just one shoe, because that's what she was wearing when she discovered that her groom had abandoned her. Miss Havisham is the epitome of a person who is stuck emotionally and spiritually. Unable to process her pain and move through it, she becomes frozen in her grief, which ripples out in bitterness to those around her. In contrast, we are called as Christians to allow God to lead us gently through seasons of suffering and into new seasons of hope.

Having been called to a vocation as a cancer patient, the time came to return again to my vocation as a vicar, and I felt keenly the emotional complexity of preparing for this change. From a time of significant hibernation, I would soon be called again into a very upfront and public ministry, which felt daunting. As I began to turn up at church events, I noticed within myself a weird mix of joy and nervousness at engaging with people again and trying to establish a new normal in our relationships, after the time when I'd largely been out of circulation.

I returned to work very gradually, grateful for the flexibility that I was given by the diocesan leadership and the parish to keep listening to my body and to keep my commitments flexible in the early months of my return. I especially enjoyed the wise advice from a nonagenarian in the parish, who encouraged me not to return before I was definitely ready, not least because 'St Mary's will be here long after we are all gone!'

I was put onto four different long-term medications in order to try to prevent the cancer from returning, and their side effects weren't easy to manage. It felt frustrating to recognize that I might never again have the energy levels that I'd had before cancer, and complicated to find my way into a new normal in terms of my physical and mental capacity. Although my return to work felt painfully slow at times, the parish were constantly loving and gracious as they continued to allow me to do as much as I could, and to cover the areas that I couldn't yet manage.

Everyone wanted to know if the cancer had gone, and I realized that people were expecting me to say that I was cancer-free. Although this was the medical opinion at that stage (my chemotherapy and radiotherapy had been to try to prevent recurrence because the cancer had been removed by the surgery), it didn't feel like the most important story to tell. I may have been officially cancer-free but I was also cancer-changed. A colleague whose wife had died within a year of a breast-cancer diagnosis said to me with thoughtful empathy, 'It changes you, doesn't it. You won't be the same after this.' In many ways I'd made peace with cancer being part of my story and my vocation, and I'd come to see it as a time of struggle and yet also of profound and unexpected blessings. It wasn't easy to try to explain all of this to those who had loved me and prayed for me through the treatment.

Everyone responded to the news that I was cancer-free with great joy and congratulations, as if I'd faced down a great enemy and come out on top, but my feelings were much more conflicted. I found the words of Dr Stevie Nash, from the TV drama *Casualty*, particularly poignant:

> Faith said to me earlier, 'Oh Stevie, you're a warrior.' And I hate that badge, because I'm not a warrior. I didn't fight cancer. I didn't beat cancer. I just survived it. And there are other women, loads of other women, who didn't win, and did that mean that they didn't fight? Does that make them not warriors? Honestly ... I don't know who I am anymore. (BBC, *Casualty*, 'Supply and Demand', Episode 2)

In the hardest days of treatment, we may long for a time when it's all over, and life can return to normal. Yet this will not be the same normal as before. We may find ourselves echoing Stevie's words, 'I don't know who I am anymore', and needing to let go of previous vocations while inviting God to lead us into new ones. As we make our emotional journey of letting go of aspects of the past and stepping forward into a different future, there may be pressure from friends, family and community that we might return to the normal that they remember. Moving into a new normal may involve grief from those around us as well as our own. This new normal will also not be static, especially as our bodies take time to heal from intense treatments and we get used to the long-term medication.

Following the Princess of Wales' long months of cancer treatment during 2024, she visited cancer centres, offering support to those undergoing treatment and sharing her story. On one visit, she talked about the difficulties of the season when the treatment is over:

> You put on a sort of brave face, stoicism through treatment. Treatment's done – then it's like 'I can crack on, get back to normal'. But actually, the phase afterwards is really difficult. You're not necessarily under the clinical team any longer, but you're not able to function normally at home as you perhaps once used to ... You have to find your new normal and that takes time. (quoted in Coughlan, 'Catherine Talks Candidly')

In the days before my penultimate chemotherapy, I faced the strange realization that in certain ways, I would miss it. The second type of chemotherapy had been so much milder for me in terms of its side effects; so each dose didn't carry such trauma. Consequently, although I knew that I wouldn't miss the chemo steroids keeping me awake, the horrible taste in my mouth all the time and the pain when they first accessed my portacath, I started thinking about the things that I would miss. I realized that I would miss the cheerful lady on the chemo ward reception, the intriguing wait to see which nurse would be looking after me each time, the joy when lunch arrived on the ward, and the very effective phlebotomy nurses who would greet me by name for the weekly blood test. A friend expressed this experience so beautifully for me:

> All the various people at chemo have become part of your support network, a valued community. And a while ago you entered this space and it was alien, and now, in a strange and complex way, you will miss all it's become for you. It's been a place where you've been cared for and where your reality has been reality – when outside you might feel alien. But despite all this, it's also a place where you know you wouldn't want to stay – this is a good and right and healthy stepping away – and as you journey on you will find new spaces and places and communities. (Revd Jane Willis)

We may be surprised by the aspects of life that we can resume easily, as well as those which will be forever changed. Others may ask us how our recovery is going, but it might be hard to identify the boundary between illness and recovery with long-term conditions requiring long-term medication. Karen O'Donnell's research into those who've experienced trauma found some illuminating things about the use of the word recovery.

> People who've experienced trauma ... felt that the word 'recovery' placed quite a heavy burden on them to be better, to be back to how they were before. Something had happened, and 'recovery' has ... a kind of bring back to the present what was lost; so it's got this kind of backward sense to it. For about a decade I've used the term 'Post-traumatic re-making'. (O'Donnell, Sofa Sunday Podcast)

O'Donnell's research reinforces the importance of not feeling the need to look backwards to try to re-establish the old normal, but rather to look forwards and allow a new normal to emerge. As we offer this re-making process to God, it can become a beautiful and creative opportunity to allow God to call us into the future, seeking God's call to us as we enter into a new season in faith and discipleship.

In his book *Recovery*, Dr Gavin Francis reflects on the difference between recovery processes that can be seen, and those that can't:

> With a limb it seemed possible to objectify the part that needed recovery, to look down on the leg and say 'that's the problem, right there'. Working to build up the leg was effortful but also visual, my progress inscribed in the bulk of my thigh, the colour of my skin, the comparison with the healthy leg at its side. My recovery from Meningitis was far more difficult to grasp, the edges of what recovery meant were far less clear. A languorous fuzzy-headed exhaustion dominated my days, burnishing the world with the bright haze of a dream or a hallucination. My body was in convalescence, but the process itself felt disembodied, ethereal, as much mental as physical. (Francis, *Recovery*, p. 6)

Our recovery, or re-making, from cancer treatment won't always be visible, or easy to quantify, and it may be hard when we're longing to see progress and improvement but there's nothing to see. Indeed, we may get worse before we get better, as our body processes the invasive treatments, and this can be especially hard.

In the First Book of Kings, Chapter 19, we find Elijah on the verge of emotional and physical collapse. Under threat from Queen Jezebel, he runs for his life, initially with his servant, but then he leaves his servant behind in Beersheba, and goes on for a further day into the desert. Here, alone and overwhelmed, Elijah prays that he might die, saying, 'I have had enough, Lord ... Take my life' (1 Kings 19.4). There in the desert God ministers to him. Elijah sleeps and then is awoken by an angel, encouraging him to eat (19.5). Having eaten, he lies down again to sleep, and then a second time, an angel meets him and encourages him to eat (19.7). In order to receive the physical, emotional and spiritual restoration that he needs, Elijah cries out to God from the solitude of the desert, and God begins to restore him through the basic necessities of rest and food. It's significant that this pattern of rest and food needed to be repeated twice, at the invitation of an angel of God. God's gracious restoration in Elijah's life took time and couldn't be rushed, and our re-making will also take time and may not be at the pace that we might hope.

Some of us won't ever be cancer-free, following a diagnosis of metastatic or stage-four cancer, but with ever-improving medical interventions, we may continue to live well for many years. Being able to live confidently against the backdrop of constant intensive treatment to try to prevent the cancer from growing further is very hard, as my friend Kate explains:

> Another Thursday, another round of chemo ... Today is cycle 130 apparently ... There is no escaping it, no getting away from it. It's always there ... in the background, poking me, like a tiny stone in your shoe ... My body is tired, tired of fighting the side effects of the drugs, tired of hurting, tired of being tired ...

Living with cancer that can never be fully removed is another emotionally complex new normal, bringing with it a particular burden of grief and fear, but also the invitation to continue to find God in the journey.

When a friend was diagnosed with a brain tumour, she got to know another local lady, of a similar age, with a similar tumour. While my friend is now doing well, the other lady's cancer is now terminal, and this kind of experience is so common on the cancer journey. The painful 'why me?' of getting cancer becomes a guilty 'why me?' when we recover and others don't. It is increasingly acknowledged that the psychological experience of 'survivor's guilt' also applies to those who have had cancer. Having joined a community of cancer patients, we may feel guilty because our cancer was caught earlier than others, or that ours is curable, while other people's can't be cured. Angela Long, who is the founder and creator of Breast Investigators, writes:

> While there is growing attention paid to our experiences as cancer survivors, there is little acknowledgment of survivor's guilt. It is neither well understood nor adequately discussed ... Survivor's guilt is often understood to be a very specific emotional response to the specific act of out-surviving others. In reality, cancer survivors experience guilt for reasons that extend far beyond simply surviving cancer when others have not. (Long, 'Survivor's Guilt')

Long goes on to acknowledge many different ways that cancer patients can feel guilty, such as the impact on our families (including genetic issues that may be passed on), having easier side effects than others and feeling permanently obliged to 'be there' for those who were there for us during treatment.

Chapter 12 of the Book of Acts is a popular passage to encourage prayer, because it tells the story of Peter's miraculous escape from prison, and how he disturbed a meeting of those praying for his rescue. It is less often noticed that, at the beginning of the chapter, King Herod 'had James, the brother of John, put to death with the sword' (v. 2). Peter and James were both key leaders in the early church, yet Peter was miraculously saved while James was killed by Herod. I wonder if Peter had survivor's guilt, as he pondered why his life was saved when his brother in Christ had been executed. Peter continued to serve the church faithfully for another 20 years, until he too was martyred.

There was a season when my vocations as a working vicar and as a cancer patient sat very closely side by side, as I straddled ongoing medical appointments with beginning to return to work. Living in the complexity of my vocations within these two very different spheres felt complicated yet beautiful, and there was something profound about living them out in parallel. During one week, I conducted two funerals, including one for a man not much older than me who had died of cancer, and then the following day I returned to the hospital to be given two new treatments intended to stop *my* cancer from returning. Being both a priest and a patient, offering care to the bereaved and then receiving care from my own medical teams, became a profound juxtaposition of the fullness of humanity and my own place of both giving and receiving within it.

As we allow our new normal to emerge, we may find our faith also changing. We may find that the ways that we used to relate to God no longer seem relevant, and patterns of prayer or styles of worship no longer seem to feed us. As we have allowed our cancer journey to be vocational, God may have broken out of the tidy boxes that we'd previously put him into in our minds, giving us a larger and deeper perspective on life and faith. As our schedules begin to be full of normal activities again, rather than medical appointments, we may find ourselves longing to stay close to God amidst the busyness. A verse from the Song of Songs felt especially relevant for me at this time: 'Who is this coming up from the wilderness, leaning on her beloved?' (Song of Songs 8.5). I found myself longing that the deep work that God had done in me through the cancer journey wouldn't be forgotten as I emerged into my busy life again. I wanted to lean on God as I emerged from my cancer wilderness, grateful for all the ways that God had held me and loved me, and living out all the things that he had taught me.

Afterword

I want to end by acknowledging again that a cancer journey is really hard. The particular nuances of struggle will be different for each of us, according to our circumstances and our cancer, but it's never easy when cancer enters our life.

Suffering and grief will always be part of our story as Christians, living in a broken and sin-drenched world, but also because we are people called and formed by the death of Christ. As we respond to Christ's invitation to follow him, sometimes our following will mean that we too need to take up our cross. Yet we are also people who know that suffering will not have the final word. There is another chapter in the story of God, a chapter filled with hope, joy and healing, and confirmed for us through the resurrection of Jesus from the dead.

I've always loved the hymn 'I cannot tell' by W. Y. Fullerton written in *c.*1920. It holds in beautiful tension the things that we don't know or understand, alongside the things that we can trust in and rely on.

I cannot tell why he, whom angels worship,
should set his love upon the sons of men,
or why, as Shepherd, he should seek the wanderers,
to bring them back, they know not how or when.
But this I know, that he was born of Mary
when Bethl'em's manger was his only home,
and that he lived at Nazareth and laboured,
and so the Saviour, Saviour of the world, is come.

I cannot tell how silently he suffered,
as with his peace he graced this place of tears,
or how his heart upon the cross was broken,
the crown of pain to three and thirty years.
But this I know, he heals the broken-hearted
and stays our sin and calms our lurking fear
and lifts the burden from the heavy laden;
for still the Saviour, Saviour of the world is here.

I cannot tell how he will win the nations,
how he will claim his earthly heritage,
how satisfy the needs and aspirations
of east and west, of sinner and of sage.
But this I know, all flesh shall see his glory,
and he shall reap the harvest he has sown,
and some glad day his sun will shine in splendour
when he the Saviour, Saviour of the world, is known.

I cannot tell how all the lands shall worship,
when at his bidding every storm is stilled,
or who can say how great the jubilation
when every heart with love and joy is filled.
But this I know, the skies will thrill with rapture,
and myriad myriad human voices sing,
and earth to heav'n, and heav'n to earth, will answer,
'at last the Saviour, Saviour of the world, is King!'

Facing suffering brings into sharp focus the many questions that we each have about our faith, including questions about suffering. Yet in suffering we can also discover in deeper and more profound ways some of the vital truths of our faith: that we are known and loved by our creator God, that he is present with us in suffering, though we may not always recognize it, and that there is no darkness so dark that the light of Christ cannot shine into it. We can use the model of this hymn to bring before God the things that we don't know or understand, perhaps using the phrase, 'I cannot tell why …' followed by our own articulation of the truths of our faith that we have learnt to trust in, 'But this I know …'

When we allow our cancer journey to be vocational, we re-affirm our belief that God can bring good from even the darkest and most desolate experiences, just as he did on the cross. A clergy friend whose daughter, Ahava, died in the womb uses the phrase 'collateral beauty' to describe the unexpected beauty that can emerge through, and in spite of, times of desperate suffering. As we face our own suffering, we can pray with hope and anticipation that God might show us the collateral beauty that he is bringing, through our painful experiences.

In the Book of Daniel, King Nebuchadnezzar puts three followers of God, Shadrach, Meshach and Abednego, into the blazing furnace because they refuse to worship a golden idol. As they prepare for their deaths, they offer the most astonishing expression of trust in God:

> 'If we are thrown into the blazing furnace, the God we serve is able to save us from it, and he will rescue us from your hand … But even if he does not, we want you to know, O King, that we will not serve your gods or worship the image of gold you have set up.' (Daniel 3.17–18)

Trusting God even if prayers are not answered as we've hoped, even if we're not rescued, is the most profound trust. These three men are indeed protected by God from the furnace and able to walk out safely. But perhaps even more significant is the moment when King Nebuchadnezzar exclaims:

> 'Weren't there three men that we tied up and threw into the fire? … Look, I see four men walking around in the fire …' (Daniel 3.24–25)

God was present in that fiery furnace as the 'fourth man'; a faithful companion for Shadrach, Meshach and Abednego in their fear. God will be a faithful companion for us too, whatever furnaces we face in our lives.

In *Revelations of Divine Love*, God shows Julian a small hazelnut in the palm of her hand which, despite its size and frailty, represents 'all that is made'. As Julian reflects with God on the hazelnut, she comes to realize three profound truths: 'The first is that God made it. The second that God loves it. And the third, that God keeps it' (Chapter 5). In suffering we can often feel fragile and insignificant, left wondering about our meaning and place within the created order. Julian encourages us that, like the tiny hazelnut, we too are made, loved and kept by God.

Tyler Staton reflects that his own cancer journey was: 'The most difficult season I've ever lived through, and probably the most spiritually transformative ... God did not remove my illness, but he did redeem it' (Staton, 'Lessons from His Cancer Journey').

Strahan Coleman writes after his own experience of extended suffering, 'God never did tell me why I went through what I did, or why he felt quiet all those years. But he did tell me he loved me, and I learnt to accept that as enough' (Coleman, *Beholding*, Chapter 11).

For myself, I have a renewed confidence in the powerful words of Paul to the Romans:

> For I am convinced that neither death nor life, neither angels nor demons, neither the present nor the future, nor any powers, neither height nor depth, nor anything else in all creation, will be able to separate us from the love of God that is in Christ Jesus our Lord. (Romans 8.38–39)

Study Guide

There are some very sensitive and personal questions here which will need careful handling in a group context. Group leaders may want to remind participants not to feel under pressure to share more than they feel comfortable with, and the group may want to think together about who they could reach out to if things are triggered that may need further pastoral care. The group may also need to be reminded of the importance of confidentiality.

Chapter 1 – Calling

- How do you relate to the idea of having a vocation based on your baptism?
- What vocations have you lived out through your life?
- Have you offered vocations that have been very painful and costly?
- What do you think of the idea of seeing cancer treatment as a vocation?
- What helps you to be conscious of God's presence with you in each moment?

Chapter 2 – Called to tussle with suffering

- What comes to your mind when you think about suffering? What has it meant in your own experience, and in the experiences of those you're close to?
- How have you related to God during times of suffering?
- Have you experienced times when God hasn't answered your prayers as you'd hoped? How did you continue to relate to God during those times?
- Do you feel able to bring your honest feelings, including disappointment and anger, to God during difficult times?

Chapter 3 – Called to face the darkness

- What times of darkness have you faced: physical, emotional or spiritual? Have you preferred to face them directly or avoid them and not think about them?
- Has darkness always been a negative experience for you? Have you received unexpected gifts from times of darkness?
- Have you experienced a Fear of Missing Out (FOMO)?
- Have you been able to invite trusted friends or spiritual advisors to accompany you as you journey through experiences of darkness?
- What spiritual disciplines have sustained you during dark times?

Chapter 4 – Called to vulnerability

- What situations have you faced that made you feel particularly vulnerable?
- Has vulnerability seemed to draw you closer to God or further away?
- Do you relate to Nouwen's idea of having within you 'a lion and a lamb'? How do you ensure that both parts of you are honoured?
- What moments of Jesus' vulnerability are particularly important for you? Could you take some time to reflect on them prayerfully in relation to your own experience of vulnerability?

Chapter 5 – Called to community

- What communities do you belong to and what do you value within them?
- During suffering, have you noticed yourself needing more time alone or more time with others? How have you been able to ask for and access what you need?
- How has the body of Christ supported you during difficult times?
- What has been your experience of reaching out and asking for help? Do you find it hard to do?

Chapter 6 – An embodied calling

- How have you experienced your body letting you down? Have you needed to grieve as you've faced these times?
- Are you able to believe that you are 'fearfully and wonderfully made'?
- How do you use your whole body in prayer and worship? Could you explore using it in new ways?
- What does it mean to you to 'offer your souls and bodies to be a living sacrifice'?

Chapter 7 – Called to be ready to die

- How do you relate to the idea of being ready to die? Have you thought about your own death?
- How have you received God's holistic healing in your life?
- How do you pray for those who are ill? How do you prefer to be prayed for when you're ill?
- What do you imagine heaven is like? What might help you to live out Billy Graham's words: 'My home is in heaven. I'm just passing through this world'?

Chapter 8 – Called to a new normal

- What seasons of change have you faced in your life, and how have you been aware of God leading you through them?
- Have you faced times of needing to let go of one vocation in order to follow God into a new one?
- What has been your experience of recovery, and how do you relate to Karen O'Donnell's idea of seeing it as 're-making'?
- Have you related to God differently during different seasons in your life?

References and Further Reading

Brother Lawrence, 1981, *The Practice of the Presence of God*, translated by E. M. Blaiklock, Hodder and Stoughton.

Brown Taylor, Barbara, 2015, *Learning to Walk in the Dark*, Canterbury Press.

Budde, Bishop Mariann Edgar, 'How We Learn to be Brave', *The Theology Network*, https://www.youtube.com/watch?v=xibt-47wN28&t=12s, accessed 7.2.2026.

Cancer Research UK, n.d., www.cancerresearchuk.org, accessed 7.2.2026.

Coleman, Strahan, 2023, *Beholding*, David C. Cook.

Comer, John Mark, 2023, 'Gethsemane Prayer', John Mark Comer Teachings Podcast, 1 September, https://open.spotify.com/episode/2ZUTppPzPJk2XHoCt7wWhh, accessed 7.2.2026.

Comer, John Mark, 2024, *Practising the Way*, Form.

Coughlan, Sean, 2025, 'Catherine Talks Candidly of "Life-Changing" Cancer Treatment', BBC News, 2 July, https://www.bbc.co.uk/news/articles/c6257z1w5ypo, accessed 9.2.2026.

Eareckson Tada, Joni, 2024, 'We are Image Bearers of God', Joni and Friends Online Daily Devotional, 21 January, https://joniandfriends.org/daily-devotional/we-are-image-bearers-of-god, accessed 7.2.2026.

Francis, Gavin, 2022, *Recovery: The Lost Art of Convalescence*, Profile.

Fullerton, William Young, *c.*1920, 'I Cannot Tell Why He Whom Angels Worship', https://hymnary.org/text/i_cannot_tell_why_he_whom_angels_worship, accessed 7.2.2026.

Graham, Billy, 1998, *Just as I am: The Autobiography of Billy Graham*, Harper Collins.

Graham, Ysenda Maxtone, 2025, 'Notebook', *Church Times*, 4 July.

Herrick, Vanessa, and Ivan Mann, 1998, *Jesus Wept: Reflections on Vulnerability in Leadership*, Darton, Longman & Todd.

Jobs, Steve, 2005, 'Stanford Commencement Speech', https://news.stanford.edu/stories/2005/06/youve-got-find-love-jobs-says, accessed 9.2.2026.

Julian of Norwich, 2015, *Revelations of Divine Love*, translated by Barry Windeatt, Oxford University Press.

Jung, Carl, 1961, *Memories, Dreams, Reflections*, Collins.

Legg, Steve, Allan Finnegan and Andy Kind, 2024, 'Where is God in a Terminal Cancer Diagnosis?', Premier UnBelievable Podcast, 24 March, https://www.premier.plus/unbelievable/podcasts/episodes/where-is-god-in-a-terminal-cancer-diagnosis-steve-legg-allan-finnegan-and-andy-kind, accessed 9.2.2026.

Lewis, C. S., 1940, *The Problem of Pain*, The Centenary Press.

Lewis, C. S., 1963, *A Grief Observed*, Harper San Francisco.

Long, Angela, 2014, 'Survivor's Guilt: Let Me Count the Ways', *The Oncology Nurse*, 7 (4), https://www.theoncologynurse.com/issue-archive/2014-issues/july-august-vol-7-no-4/16184-survivor-s-guilt-let-me-count-the-ways, accessed 3.5.2026.

Mackesy, Charlie, 2019, *The Boy, the Mole, the Fox and the Horse*, Penguin.

Marczewski, Jane, 2021, 'God is on the Bathroom Floor', Nightbirde Blog, https://www.nightbirde.co/blog/2021/9/27/god-is-on-the-bathroom-floor, accessed 19.1.2026.

Matheson, George, 1882, 'O Love that Wilt Not Let Me Go', https://hymnary.org/text/o_love_that_wilt_not_let_me_go, accessed 26.1.2026.

McGrath, Alister, 2016, *C. S. Lewis, a Life. Eccentric Genius, Reluctant Prophet*, Tyndale House Publishers.

Moriarty, Liane, 2019, *Nine Perfect Strangers*, Penguin.

Nouwen, Henri J. M., 1996, *The Inner Voice of Love*, Bantam Doubleday Dell.

Nouwen, Henri J. M., 2009, *The Way of the Heart: The Spirituality of the Desert Fathers and Mothers*, HarperCollins.

O'Donnell, Karen, 2025, Sofa Sunday Podcast, 25 May, https://soundcloud.com/oasischurchbath/sofasundaykarenodonnell, accessed 7.2.2026.

Oliver, Mary, 2020, 'The Summer Day', in *Devotions*, Penguin.

Palmer, Parker, 1999, *Let your Life Speak: Listening for the Voice of Vocation*, Jossey-Bass.

Peterson, Eugene, 1993, *The Contemplative Pastor: Returning to the Art of Spiritual Direction*, William B. Eerdmans.

Richards, Anne, 2025, 'The Death of Us', Modern Church Blog, 25 June, https://modernchurch.org.uk/the-death-of-us, accessed 8.2.2026.

Runcorn, David, 2018, *The Language of Tears: Their gift, mystery and meaning*, Canterbury Press.

Runcorn, David, 2020, 'Reflections on the Resurrection', David Runcorn Blog, 13 April, https://davidruncorn.com/drwp/reflections-on-the-resurrection-6-6/, accessed 7.2.2026.

St John of the Cross, 2008, *Dark Night of the Soul*, translated and edited by E. Allison Peers, Wilder Publications.

Scott, David, 2016, *The Love That Made Mother Teresa*, Sophia Institute Press.

'Setting God's People Free', 2017, Church of England report, presented to General Synod, https://www.churchofengland.org/sites/default/files/2021-10/gs-misc-1302-setting-gods-people-free-update.pdf, accessed 26.1.2026.

Staton, Tyler, 2022, 'Ask, Seek, Knock (Silence and Persistence) ft. Pete Greig', Praying Like Monks, Living Like Fools Podcast, 21 November, https://podcasts.apple.com/za/podcast/ask-seek-knock-silence-and-persistence-ft-pete-greig/id1650479108?i=1000586981946, accessed 26.1.2026.

Staton, Tyler, 2022, *Praying Like Monks, Living Like Fools: An Invitation to the Wonder and Mystery of Prayer*, Hodder & Stoughton.

Staton, Tyler, 2022, 'Vocation', sermon based on Ephesians 4.1–28, 15 August, Bridgetown Church, Portland, USA, https://bridgetown.church/teachings/ephesians/vocation, accessed 26.1.2026.

Staton, Tyler, 2025, *The Familiar Stranger: (Re)Introducing the Holy Spirit to Those in Search of an Experiential Spirituality*, Hodder & Stoughton.

Staton, Tyler, 2025, 'Healing, with Mark Sayers', The Familiar Stranger Podcast, 25 March, www.youtube.com/watch?v=niCoSomOJsY, accessed 3.5.2026.

Staton, Tyler, 2025, 'Lessons from His Cancer Journey', Carey Nieuwhof Leadership Podcast, Episode 706, https://careynieuwhof.com/episode 706, accessed 26.1.2026.

Sunlife Cost of Dying Report, 2024, https://www.sunlife.co.uk/siteassets/documents/cost-of-dying/sunlife-cost-of-dying-report-2024.pdf/, accessed 1.9.2025.

Temple, William, 1934, *Nature, Man and God*, Macmillan.

Tomlinson, Jill, 2014, *The Owl Who was Afraid of the Dark*, Farshore.

Vanstone, W. H., 1982, *The Stature of Waiting*, Darton, Longman & Todd.

Volf, Miroslav, 1997, *After our Likeness: The Church as the Image of the Trinity*, William B. Eerdmans.

West, Christopher, 2003, 'Theology of the Body: An Education in Being Human', https://irp.cdn-website.com/eda845f4/files/uploaded/the-theology-of-the-body-an-education-in-being-human.pdf, accessed 9.2.2026.

Willard, Dallas, 2006, *The Great Omission: Reclaiming Jesus's Essential Teachings on Discipleship*, Monarch Books.

www.ingramcontent.com/pod-product-compliance
Lightning Source LLC
La Vergne TN
LVHW091034150826
845672LV00006BA/1817

* 9 7 8 1 7 8 6 2 2 7 4 6 1 *